Living Without Fear

Living Without Fear:

Understanding Cancer and the New Therapies

Thomas E. Wagner, Ph.D.
&
Michael J. Bugeja, Ph.D.

Whitston Publishing Company, Inc.
Albany, New York
2001

Library of Congress Control Number 2001-135033

ISBN 0-87875-526-8

Printed in the United States of America

For Tong and Diane

Table of Contents

Chapter Three

MUTANTS AND GATEKEEPERS

Chapter Four

THE TWISTED PATH FROM PRE-CANCER TO CANCER

Chapter Five

LESSONS FROM THE AIDS VIRUS

Chapter Six

TRADITIONAL THERAPY

Chapter Seven

GENE THERAPY: A GREAT YET LIMITED HOPE

Chapter Eight

IMMUNOTHERAPY: HELPING THE BODY CURE ITSELF

Chapter Nine
The New Cancer Chemotherapy

FOREWORD

Two newsworthy events occurred while we (geneticist Thomas Wagner and ethicist Michael Bugeja) were busy researching data for this book. One was a local speech by a famous orator and politician. The other was breaking news in both cancer and the publishing world. We calmly heeded these happenings and persevered, as we had been doing, for the better part of one year when we decided to halt our individual research projects and collaborate on a work that would lessen the fear of cancer and restore hope in millions worldwide.

The first news event featured an ambassador of hope, the Rev. Jesse Jackson. The famed orator was visiting Ohio University where we were teaching at the time. (Dr. Wagner has since become Director of Oncology Research at the Greenville Hospital System Cancer Treatment Center in Greenville, South Carolina, and distinguished professor of molecular medicine at Clemson University.) That night, in his typical passionate way, Jesse Jackson addressed thousands of people attending his speech in the domed basketball stadium on campus.

The Rev. Jackson asked members of the audience to stand up if they had cancer. Several dozen did. Then he asked those to stand who had family members stricken with breast and other cancers. More and more rose from their seats. Finally he asked all those present to stand if cancer had touched their lives in a substantial way. Practically everyone was standing.

Sadly, for that reason, practically everyone is a potential reader of *Living Without Fear*. Throughout this book we were careful to identify those readers: people with or at risk for cancer, the health conscious, and their loved ones. We know that dozens of cancer books have been published in recent years but none embracing all segments of the cancer saga. A full year earlier, we also knew that only a few rather scientific works focused on the molecular breakthroughs and genetic treatments that were being reported in journals or being tested in research trials. Dr. Wagner, one of the world's leading molecular geneticists, was in possession of cutting-edge information. His colleague, Michael Bugeja, was an award-winning writer, teacher, and ethicist who had a science and media background and could translate the new therapies into prose that everyone could understand. So we stopped our own research projects and went to work on what we knew would be an informative book with one goal: to eradicate fear associated with cancer and, thereby, renew hope.

Soon after Jesse Jackson spoke to the audience at Ohio University, another news story erupted nationwide, based on optimistic reports that a new cancer therapy might defeat the disease once and for all. The therapy was *angiogenesis inhibition*—the blocking of the formation of blood vessels feeding a cancerous tumor. We questioned the developing story because we knew the procedure had not yet undergone extensive clinical trials. True, angiogenesis inhibition looked and still looks promising, but we knew that Dr. Wagner had been curing tumors in mice for years via a host of different therapies, although not specifically via tumor angiogenesis. We also knew that shrinking or eradicating tumors in mice is one thing; doing so in humans is another. But the overoptimistic reports about the angiogenesis process resulted in a deluge of media coverage on cancer and the new therapies. News magazines dedicated cover stories to cancer research. Newspapers went into depth about treatment. So did network TV. All the while, clinical trials—an important component of accountable science—continued, with no immediate news about instant cancer cures. Without such cures, the media lost interest momentarily in cancer research.

This book does not offer cures. If it did, we would be guilty of raising false hope in millions of cancer patients, survivors, and their families. Yet the new emerging therapies are covered here in detail, including angiogenesis inhibition. One of the goals of the book is to educate and inform cancer patients and loved ones so that patients can acquire quality treatment. Moreover, throughout the book, we take pains to hammer home a common theme: *overcoming fear*. To help you in that endeavor, we have developed a sequence of exercises to envision cancer at the molecular level and to enhance your consciousness (and confidence) at the creative level. These powerful exercises call on readers not only to imagine the molecular and cellular landscape but also to increase their well-being by developing an improved attitude. As such, we hope to convey to readers a *wellness philosophy* based on a few universal truths in which we believe deeply.

We share a unique vision. We believe that human beings can solve any problem on earth *as long as they take the time to understand the problem* and that human beings are distinct from animals *because we can make anything we envision.* Those two attitudes have joined in what we hope is a work that will inspire, inform, and enlist you and your loved ones in the potentially winnable war against cancer.

Thomas Wagner, Ph.D.
Greer, South Carolina

Michael J. Bugeja, Ph.D.
Athens, Ohio

Chapter One

Cancer and the Wellness Process

Books must follow sciences, and not sciences books.

—Sir Francis Bacon

The book you are reading is a combination of art and science. The science, of course, came first, following the general rule of poet-scientist Sir Francis Bacon (1561-1626), father of the scientific method and oft cited as the true author of Shakespeare's dramatic works. *Living Without Fear* unravels biological rather than poetical miracles and mysteries. We hope to give you *more* than hope. We want to empower you with the fact of science and the foresight of art to help you:

- Envision the building blocks of life, so that you understand why cancer occurs.
- Imagine cancer at the molecular level, so that you grasp the origins of the disease.
- Embrace the relevance of biology and the revelations of consciousness, so that you can deploy both in the treatment and prevention of cancer.
- Consider cures now or soon available, so that you can be an informed health consumer.
- Combat the fear associated with this disease, so that you enjoy life to the fullest.

Heart disease, the leading cause of death in the United States, is not the most feared when it comes to diagnoses. That distinction is reserved for cancer. For awhile in the 1990s, the dread disease was overshadowed by AIDS; but with the advent of seemingly effective new drug therapies and faint promises of an effective vaccine in the foreseeable future, cancer has returned as our most menacing health concern.

Does cancer deserve such an ominous distinction? Like other facets of this disease, the answer is complicated. Certainly, cancer is the most fundamentally complex disorder facing today's medical research community. Essentially it disrupts one of the most basic functions of the entire life process, and the ravaging effects of its progression in an advanced cancer patient is as, or more, devastating than any other life-threatening disease.

These facts alone play on our fears of a cancer diagnosis. But indeed, there is more than hope on the medical horizon. Monumental strides have been made over the last several years, especially in our understanding of cancer at the molecular level. We know more about the mechanisms that trigger the disease and how it can progress toward its final, life-threatening conclusion. Such knowledge has led the medical community to a myriad of new and potentially powerful modes of treatment—many of which will no longer have the devastating side-effects of current treatments like chemotherapy. Accompanying these innovative approaches are methods to prevent both the onset and

> **❖ Inspiration Point**
>
> **New treatments on the horizon will no longer have the devastating side-effects of radiation and chemotherapy.**

pathways of this disease. However, to take full advantage of modern-day science, cancer patients and their loved ones need to know about these new treatments and prevention techniques. As you might imagine, knowledge is at the crux of combating this illness and providing you with *knowledge* is the objective of this book.

❧ ❧ ❧

Knowledge Lessens Fear

Knowledge, as the saying goes, is power. But knowledge can also help you overcome fear. And the power of the mind can aid the healing process, as any doctor who has prescribed a placebo can attest. So, in a real sense, this book represents a kind of "therapy for the mind" of those afflicted with cancer and "antidote for the soul" of loved ones who carry with them fear's burden and baggage. In addition, for those without cancer, the best defense to ward off cancer is insight into how to prevent it from occurring in the first place. So *Living Without Fear* is also written for the person interested in wellness.

We believe that a more detailed understanding of the cancer process—especially at the molecular level—affords a patient a much stronger feeling of involvement in his or her treatment. Here's why. Consider what you know about a simple injury—a scratch, say, on your fingertip. You may be annoyed at the pain or inconvenience; but you're fairly sure how to treat the wound by bandaging it and applying a salve. You know that by doing this the healing process will soon take hold, especially if you keep the cut clean to avoid infection. If the cut doesn't scab and begin to heal in a few days, you will know something is amiss and probably will see the doctor. That's a simple comparison, of course; cuts, even infected ones, are rarely life-threatening. But the comparison is apt when it comes to a person's *awareness* and *state of mind.* The cut that won't heal is a signal of a serious problem. There are signals for cancer, too, only they occur at the cellular level. That's why it's important to know the process and progression of cancer at that level. Similarly, understanding cancer—its therapies and prevention—can give a patient a greater sense of self-involvement during a personal time of physical and emotional upheaval. Through the mind, you reclaim at least some of the control that fear has usurped from you. In fact, being able to visualize how therapy can inhibit or terminate the cancer process can spur in the patient a genuine sense of power—power over a disease that intends to rob one of that very feeling.

> **❖ Inspiration Point**
>
> **Visualizing effective treatment can bestow in you a sense of power over a disease that intends to rob you of that very feeling.**

❧ ❧ ❧

Mind and Medicine

If you doubt the power of the mind in treating and preventing cancer, you forfeit one more weapon in your war against this merciless killer. To respect the mind, consider the biological "miracle" of the human body, Nature's most complex machine, with voluntary functions (holding hands, for instance) and involuntary ones like breathing or blinking. Add to this the concept of "consciousness," a still-mysterious aspect of the brain, the *soul* (if you are religious), and then you may realize, as Shakespeare did: "What a piece of work is man! how infinite in faculty! in form, in moving, how express and admirable! in action how like an angel! in apprehension how like a god!" One finds the same sense of awe in Charles Darwin, the great scientist of evolution. True, he acknowledged that our origins were "lowly," rather than bestowed instantaneously by God. But he also spoke about "[m]an with all his noble qualities . . . with his god-like intellect which has penetrated into the movements and constitution of the solar system. . . ." Now, at the dawn of a new millenium, we not only can see with space telescopes to the edges of the universe; we also can envision the microscopic systems of the cell. Increasingly the medical community is acknowledging the power of the mind, especially with respect to stress-reducing meditation (or even prayer) as a partner in the healing process.

> **❖ Inspiration Point**
>
> **Increasingly, prayer and meditation are being accepted as partners in the healing process, along with surgical and pharmaceutical intervention.**

Meditation, spiritual or secular, is a practice not consigned to any one religion or culture—but something viewed as globally true. For instance, even in the non-theistic tradition of Buddhism, practitioners meditate to ease illness or improve health. Increasingly in North America, spiritual and/or prayerful meditation is being accepted as a partner in the healing process, along with surgical and pharmaceutical intervention. Prayer, in particular, seems to affect stress hormones, leading to lower blood pressure and easier breathing, for instance. In a recent *Time Magazine* article, David Felten, chairman of the Department of Neurobiology at the University of Rochester, says, "Anything involved with meditation and controlling the state of mind that alters hormone activity has the potential to have an impact on the immune system." Of course, this is not news to the typical layperson. A 1998 Time/CNN poll reported that 82% of respondents believed in the power of prayer. "[I]f we paid attention to our patients," says physician Tony Rippo of the Sante Fe Institute for Medicine and Prayer, "maybe we would hear that they want doctors to treat the whole person."

We agree.

❧ ❧ ❧

Enhancing the Healing Process

We want to add two other powerful elements to the healing triangle of surgical, pharmaceutical and meditative intervention: a cellular vantage point and an ethical viewpoint. We hope to *renew* hope with this book because, like Darwin and Shakespeare, we believe in the dual miracle of body and mind. We also believe that cancer patients and their loved ones seek information about their illness, especially if that information can help in their own treatment. But many doctors withhold technical explanations from patients, especially about the happenings at the cellular level. This is where cancer sets up camp and support systems to execute its potentially lethal functions. You'll learn those explanations here.

You'll also learn that if the mind can move mountains, it can nudge a molecule—theoretically, at least. Although cancer is complex and powerful, it is *not* as complex as the mind nor as powerful as consciousness. When we are conscious, we are aware. When we know about treatments, we can make more confident decisions. And we can harness the mind to enhance treatment or the healing process.

A case in point: In a classic experiment, patients suffering from severe stomach ulcers were provided with tablets containing a micro-monitor for acidity. This tiny probe reported the acid levels from within a patient's stomach by sending radio signals to a visual display unit outside of the body. Without such a display unit, the patient would never know about high acid levels—except via *pain*, the body's natural signal that something is wrong internally. But as long as the patients in this experiment could observe their acid levels and monitor internal changes in those levels, they were able to effectively control their stomach acid *and* their ulcers.

Unfortunately, it is not possible to provide a cancer patient with a monitor showing the growth rate of his or her tumor. Nonetheless, a patient *can* monitor the process of tumor development and *visualize treatment at the cellular level*—the life-death battleground of cancer. At the end of each chapter, there are "Envisioning Exercises," helping you "see" the proteins, molecules and genes associated with each chapter topic. You will use artistic techniques to aid you in this process and will create, the way artists do—by writing, drawing, or just plain imagining—to help alleviate stress, fear and bestow a feeling of attainment. We know that reducing stress and fear and experiencing the euphoria of creation may not reverse symptoms of cancer—nor are the benefits of monitoring tumor growth and visualizing treatment yet proven, in the strictest scientific sense. But in increasing numbers, many doctors and scientists believe that patients who can envision the cellular battlefield can spot "enemy" columns of cancer and wage a strategic war against them, aiding the healing process.

❧ ❧ ❧

Uniting Body and Mind

Much of the technical information in this book comes not from the clinic, but from the research laboratory. Thus, this book is an attempt to describe the molecular events leading to cancer and to explain the disease in clear, crisp terminology. The simplest definition of cancer is a disruption in the body's ability to control the replication of cells. Before a cell dies, it copies itself. This happens continuously in the body—one of its many miracles—replacing the physical you, literally, with new life. But cancer strikes when a cluster (or clusters) of certain cells go out-of-control, replicating themselves over and over again like renegades, able to elude some of the body's natural defense mechanisms and eventually infiltrating, overcoming and conquering inner terrain—your lungs, your liver, your colon. To understand cancer, its treatment and prevention, one needs to understand:

- ❖ How these renegade cells avoid an army of natural safeguards that would block their uncontrolled expansion.
- ❖ How the ensuing initial tumor is able to sustain itself, getting enough nutrition to allow its continued growth.
- ❖ How the tumor is able to spread or metastasize to distant sites within the body.

The early chapters address these issues. But, as we said, cancer is complex. So answers to these questions are often different for each type of cancer, making this not truly a disease but a *class* of diseases. That's why cancer is humankind's most feared mortal enemy. In combating it, we need not only the world's best oncologists, laboratories, hospitals, clinics, and pharmaceutical companies, but also patients and loved ones who want to prevent cancer's occurrence or recurrence and help the afflicted seek effective treatment.

Before the advent of the biotechnology revolution, studies aimed at developing therapies for cancer patients consisted mainly of randomly testing chemical agents and ionizing radiation for their ability to kill tumor cells. Admittedly, past and much of present-day cancer therapy was and is based upon the results of these older studies. The good news is that a whole new class of cancer therapies now emerging will likely dominate future cancer treatments—all a result of the contemporary approach to cancer research which is based on understanding the molecular conditions that allow the disease to begin and progress. This offers hope and optimism for the effective treatment of some cancers now and perhaps all aspects of this class of disease in the near future. To comprehend that future, and act on it as soon as possible, you need to understand the logic behind new therapies and those soon to become available. They are described in the latter chapters.

> **❖ Inspiration Point**
>
> **A whole new class of cancer therapies is rapidly becoming available. To take full advantage of them, you should know the logic behind them and empower yourself with information.**

Indeed, *Living Without Fear* was written to muster readers into the ranks of cancer researchers who know that only by understanding exactly how this cellular aberration begins and persists will we ever hope to interfere with its progression and effect a cure. Again, this book does not offer a cure. But it does offer more than peace of mind: it offers the *power of mind* to know cancer and to join in active participation—regardless of your condition, general health, or area of expertise—to obliterate the fear associated with this illness.

We are certain of this: one day, sooner rather than later, we will all hear good news about cancer. We won't hear the dire prognoses of the doctor's office accompanied by the hopeless weeping of loved ones. We'll hear this: the disease's own death-knell, assuring a better future for us and for generations to follow. Conversely, we also understand that cancer patients and/or loved ones are more interested in the present than in the future. So are medical consumers—people at risk of contracting cancer and those interested in wellness and cancer prevention. So before embarking on our cellular journey, we will sate that thirst for information by making specific recommendations for each of our readers.

❧ ❧ ❧

What You Can Do *Now*

We believe that understanding cancer can allay fear and that a positive attitude will arise from the absence of fear. We believe that liberation from the bonds of fear empowers the cancer patient and his or her loved ones to join the physician and the scientist in combating this disease. We also believe that understanding the cancer process—the interplay among life's molecules and mutations—is vital now more than ever because of new molecular weapons in the war against cancer. Those weapons can explode the myth of cancer's invincibility and liberate us from our fear of this disease. We'll explore more about these weapons in upcoming chapters. For now, heed the guidelines below, addressing the cancer patient, the person with high-risk factors for contracting cancer, the health conscious individual who wishes to protect himself or herself from cancer, and those who love and care for people of these three groups.

✔ For The Cancer Patient

Many cancer patients may feel doubly unfortunate. You not only have been diagnosed with cancer, you've been diagnosed just before the advent of a whole new era of more effective cancer therapy. However, you shouldn't feel left out. Again, this is a matter of attitude and perception akin to seeing a glass half filled with hope, or half empty. With each passing day the prognosis for almost all cancer patients is better. Better yet, there are actions you, as a cancer patient, can choose to take that will further improve your individual situation.

First and foremost, learn as much as possible about the molecular and cellular aspects of your specific disease. While cancer patients usually try to understand their life-threatening illness, they often fail to recognize their disorder at the level of the organs and tissues of their body. Doing that requires a cellular vision.

We will help give you such a vision. You will know that cancer is not a disease of organs or tissues but an assault upon the much more microscopic cellular and molecular land- and seascapes of these structures. It is virtually impossible for anyone to apprehend cancer or the cancer process without a basic understanding of cellular and molecular biology. By reading this book, you will develop such an understanding and be proud of it! Only a few years ago the most accomplished scientists and physicians in the world did not know the fundamentals of innovative cancer treatments and strategies. Only a few decades ago cancer patients routinely were not informed that they had a life-threatening illness. You will know your illness on the cellular level. And while your specific type of cancer may not be mentioned in this book, you will better know how to ask questions and solicit pertinent information, delving into the depths of the molecular and cellular topography of your own personal enemy. The key to gaining a true sense of your enemy is to know as much as possible about the specific molecular origins of your cancer and the path it has taken through the cellular topography of your tissues. When you do, you will envision the battlefield of your natural defensive armies and navies. Many of the actions you can take via your personal physician or surgeon to maximize your chances against your disease stem from this knowledge of your cancer. So familiarize yourself with both research related to the treatment of your disease and ongoing clinical trials of new treatments for your disease. And if you are limited because of your condition, ask a loved one to assist you.

Personal research is also empowerment. As you study your disease in greater depth, the names of those scientists who specialize in your particular form of cancer will become familiar to you. Although cancer research is usually published in highly technical journals found only in medical libraries, more and more abstracts of such research can be found on the internet and are available to anyone with computer access. Each day new databases become available. Each month computer access improves. A few years ago, such research could be done only in large public or university libraries. Now even remote rural ones have computer access. Utilize this resource, or ask a loved one to do so on your behalf.

> ❖ **Inspiration Point**
>
> **You should approach your therapy as an elite athlete approaches training sessions or workouts, not as a drudgery to be endured, but as an opportunity to improve.**

Using the internet is also a wonderful way to keep abreast of the ongoing cancer clinical trials throughout the United States and the world. An updated listing, categorized by the specific cancer targeted in the clinical trial, is provided by the National Cancer Institute's web site (www.nci.nih.gov). Early knowledge of clinical trials—for which you might even qualify, although conditions and candidates are heavily screened—can be located at this site or via the links posted.

Fully participate in and invest your energy, belief, and faith in your current treatment. While it may or may not cure you it could well sustain you until a time when more effective modes of treatment are available. Finally, while we believe that learning as much as possible about your disease is of utmost importance, this quest should never intrude upon or impede the primary role of the cancer patient, namely: *to engage in your therapy to the fullest extent possible.*

In that regard, here's a suggestion: You should approach your therapy as an elite athlete approaches training sessions or workouts, not as a drudgery to be endured, but as an opportunity to improve. The healthier the patient, the more effective the therapy. Live as healthy a life as possible, paying attention to diet, prescribed medication, and anything else that your physician or surgeon recommends. By participating in this manner, you can also improve your own sense of well being, along with developing a more positive attitude. Physicians now agree the greater your vitality, energy, and physiological condition, the more active your immune system can become.

> **❖ Inspiration Point**
>
> **Forget about finding a cure *today*. Strive to live today and tomorrow as healthy as possible. Now is the time *to buy time* . . . until the new therapies come on line.**

You will understand the importance of the immune system as you read upcoming chapters. You should follow specific exercise and dietary recommendations from your doctor, who knows you and your condition best, especially if you are undergoing chemotherapy. Those who have the opportunity to join an immunotherapy cancer trial should be doubly conscious of this recommendation. The fact that you are a cancer patient is no excuse to live in an unhealthy way. At this stage in your life is it more important than ever to maintain the highest standards of diet, exercise, and good general health.

Attitude is vital now, also. Don't lose hope. While no one knows for sure, scientists may be on the verge of conquering cancer in general and your disease in particular. Don't worry so much about achieving a cure *today*, but aim at getting to tomorrow as healthy as possible, and to the next week, the next month, and the next year. Now is the time *to buy time* . . . until the new therapies come on line. Keep yourself strong enough to participate in these new therapies. This is not false hope, but genuine hope. Today hope has a face: that of gene therapy, immunotherapy, and new age chemotherapy. We will delve into all of these areas of hope in this book.

✔ For Those at Risk

Those at risk for cancer should carefully read this book to understand the disease at the molecular and cellular levels. That will help you make intelligent health-care choices in the years ahead. In fact, it is almost *more* important for people at risk for a specific cancer to learn about the disease that threatens them. If you have risk factors for colorectal cancer, become an expert on it. Learn not only about new therapies coming on line but also about preventative measures you can take such as scheduling regular rectal exams and eating a high fiber diet. Regular exams can identify polyps that can then be easily removed before they endanger you. A high fiber diet scours away the "sticky" cells of the intestine before they can become polyps, one of the early steps on the long, twisted path toward cancer, explained in detail later. If you are at risk for other cancers, learn as much as you can about your disease on the internet, from your physician, and from the American Cancer Society. You can contact the agency at (www.cancer.org) or by telephone toll-free at 1-800-ACS-2345.

If you are at risk, keep yourself at the peak of health—according to a program prescribed by your physician. Exercise probably will play a key role in that program, as well as diet. You also know the importance of the immune system and how exercise and good diet enhance it. The immune system is one of your most

> ❖ **Inspiration Point**
>
> **Although no one can promise that you will not contract cancer, envision yourself in the group of those with risk factors *who will not contract cancer.***

essential weapons to resist the progress of any cancer. Remember, time may favor you because cancer evolves via a long and complex pathway after the initial mutation. And mutations, you will realize, are nothing to fear. They happen in all of us. The healthier you are and the stronger your immune system, the better you will be able to naturally block an early step in the particular cancer process.

Health includes attention to diet. Ask your personal physician to recommend an anti-cancer diet. You may have seen public service announcements from the American Cancer Society suggesting a daily diet consisting of at least five fruits and vegetables. Fruits and vegetables sound healthy, but why are they cancer preventative foods? The agents in our environment and in many of our cooked foods that cause mutations are most reactive with DNA in the form of free radicals. A free radical is an atom or atom group with an unpaired electron that reacts with a cell, causing cellular or genetic damage. The natural vitamins and anti-oxidants found in fresh fruits and vegetables deactivate free radicals and may well reduce the incidence of mutation in our DNA. We cannot totally stop mutation, but we can perhaps reduce its incidence. You can do that by reducing factors that might initiate the cancer process, including the frequency of its progression by way of accumulated mutations. Diet can certainly help in this mission. So can mental attitude. Although no one can promise that you will not contract cancer, envision yourself in the group of those with risk factors who *will not contract cancer*. At the very least, that mindset will keep you motivated.

✔ For The Health Conscious

If you haven't done so already, read the previous sections of this chapter, even if you are not a cancer patient or face an increased risk of becoming one. In addition:

- ❖ Understand cancer at the molecular and cellular level by carefully reading up-coming chapters.
- ❖ Maintain a vigorous immune system by shunning tobacco products, avoid being overweight, exercise regularly, and follow a healthy diet.

> **❖ Inspiration Point**
>
> **Look forward to regular checkups, knowing early detection of any disease increases your chances of beating the disease.**

Before losing weight and/or adopting an exercise plan and diet, consult your physician. And that, alas, is your most important step—have regular checkups. Don't fear checkups. Look forward to them, knowing that early detection of any disease often can lead to effective treatment.

To keep a positive attitude, celebrate your own values about the importance of health awareness. Keep reading and learning about cancer and health care and even participate by donating funds or time to hospitals, clinics, and research facilities, or to causes promoted by the American Cancer Society. Pass along your values about health awareness whenever possible and enlist others in the campaign, not only in the crusade against cancer, but also in the fight against *fear*.

✔ For Loved Ones

We end this chapter with a special message to you. Love is an ethical concept as mysterious and intricate as the cell. There is no real evolutionary reason for love because lust alone would propagate the species. Love is not survival of the fittest but compassion for the *unfit*. Love is commitment and involves participation—in health care and lifestyle issues, certainly, but also in hobbies, causes, and passions. Love also is "sacrifice" in the truest sense of that ancient word, for when a person you love becomes ill or experiences pain, you want to bear that burden. As some ethicists argue, love has a philosophical "opposite," and it is *not* hate. Love and hate, in fact, are close cousins because they often evoke passionate emotions. The opposite of love is *fear*.

Fear is not so mysterious. There is a real evolutionary reason for fear because it generates the "fight or flight" response, enabling species to defend or protect themselves. Fear is about survival. It lacks compassion for the unfit because it is concerned about self-preservation or self-interest, from protecting one's turf to protecting one's feelings. Fear is lack of commitment and avoidance of participation. It certainly isn't "sacrifice" when a loved one has cancer, is at a risk for cancer, or is concerned about getting cancer. Fear deafens when doctors speak. Fear overlooks wellness and cancels appointments with physicians. Fear is indifferent to anyone else's concerns, and as such, ruins attitudes—not only for the person doing the fearing—but for loved ones as well.

> **❖ Inspiration Point**
>
> **Your attitude is as important as ever to a loved one facing the challenges of cancer. *That person knows you on the basis of love rather than fear.***

Conversely, fear is only natural when the health of someone we cherish is at stake. You have to face your situation just as your loved one may be facing his or hers, and realize this: *Fear has no place in the fight against cancer.* Fear changes people precisely when others need them most. Now more than ever your loved one may need your research, your compassion, your participation, and your sacrifice—putting your life on hold for awhile, perhaps, while facing the challenges of the day, knowing you have the inner resources to meet some if not all of them.

In China, there is a loving ethical concept called Jen (pronounced *"ZHUN"*). It is the practice of perfect kindness and includes "a harmony of viewpoints," seeing your loved one as he or she wishes to be seen, doing for others as you wish done for you, and, most importantly, counting the day's blessings, from the beauty of sunrise to the whisper of willows, to the texture of silk, to the taste of peeled orange, to the smell of its rind. So our recommendation to you is to practice Jen in all of your dealings, especially with loved ones.

Your attitude is as important as ever to a loved one facing the challenges of cancer. That person knows you on the basis of love rather than fear. To offset cancer's effect on you, note the many kind acts that happen during the day. You will be surprised to learn that many more kind acts occur than you might imagine. Keep a kindness journal and record each kind act and how that has affected your attitude. Gauge how your own kindness has helped a loved one or enhanced interactions with those caring for your loved one. Remember that you will apt to be most *unkind* when you are busy, and coping with the illnesses of others will keep you busier than ever. However, be sure to take time out during the day to enjoy its many blessings, according to the tenets of Jen.

Kindness may not restore health but it usually quells fear and replenishes love. As you will learn in this book, *there are gatekeepers of the soul as well as of the cell, and kindness is chief among them.*

✔ For All—Envisioning Exercises

At the end of each chapter you will encounter envisioning exercises. A primary objective of this book is to hone the mind and expand consciousness. That is what the envisioning exercises are designed to help do. By doing these envisioning exercises, you will experience a deeper level of wellness. Many are designed to lessen fear. They also aim to sharpen your vision at the cellular level, where cancer occurs. You'll also learn about ethical concepts like courage and commitment. That, too, will enhance your attitude. As your knowledge grows, so will your confidence and consciousness, your allies in the war against cancer.

❦ ❦ ❦

Envisioning Exercise

Solitary Meditation

Objective: To experience a sense of relaxation, well-being and less fear.

Where: A quiet place where you are alone and will not be disturbed. This can be a study, a special place, in a park, or in a hospital chapel. Most importantly a place without television, radio, telephone or the possibility of untimely intrusion.

How often: Twice a day to once a week—but really as often as you'd like.

Below are seven easy steps to help you develop a sense of relaxation, well-being, and experience less fear. As part of this meditation you'll be re-envisioning an act of kindness. Before you begin to meditate, read over the steps several times so that you know the basic technique.

1. *Find a quiet place to meditate.* Do this exercise when you are least likely to be disturbed.

2. *Before you begin, take a deep breath or a few deep breaths.* Get comfortable in a sitting or reclining position . . . and feel relaxed.

3. *Close your eyes to enhance your inner vision.* Meditation often begins with a deep breath and closed eyes. Poets and other artists often close their eyes not so much to call forth the "muse" but to envision aspects of their work with a clear picture in the mind. If you are unexpectedly interrupted, *be kind,* as kindness is a focus of this particular exercise.

4. *Imagine a black, blank movie screen.* This blankness may be hard to achieve at first. Take your time. If images pop up on the "screen" of your mind, gently push them out. Just relax and breathe deeply and regularly.

5. *Remember an act of kindness that somehow impacted your life.* It could have been a parent, surprising you with compassion when you anticipated anger. It could have been a teacher inspiring you to take a different view or path in life. It could have been a complete stranger—some modern-day good Samaritan who seemingly appeared out of nowhere. We all have experienced many acts of kindness that have impacted our lives. Pick one.

6. *Hone in on the specific act of kindness as if you were reliving that moment again.* Remember smells. Textures. Sights. All the details of the experience to stimulate your senses.

7. *Now concentrate on a single gesture, feeling, facial expression or action that you remember at the precise moment of kindness.* Freeze that image as if your mind were a camera taking a snapshot. Then imagine how an artist

might draw or sculpt that ending image. How would a musician intone it on a piano or other instrument? How would a dancer represent it on stage? How would a storyteller, poet, or writer on the page?

Imagine these scenarios to utilize your innate creativity and fully experience a relaxed state of well-being and reduced level of fear.

Chapter Two

The Life Process and Origins of Cancer

We have only to believe. And the more threatening and irreducible reality appears, the more firmly and desperately must we believe. Then, little by little, we shall see the universal horror unbend, and then smile upon us, and then take us in its more than human arms.

—Pierre Teilhard de Chardin (1881-1955)

Consider, for a moment, something beautiful: an elaborate Japanese origami, those lovely multifolded paper creations of, say, a blossom or an animal. You can marvel at the craft of origami-making; but it is difficult to mimic without carefully observing how the creation unravels from the folds of a small square of colored paper. Life, of course, is a beautiful creation—vastly more complex than origami. But life also unfolds, and understanding the process will reveal something to you about the origins of cancer. Unfortunately many students of the life process, particularly in medicine, only look at life from birth to death. The beginnings of life are just as marvelous and enlightening to behold, especially life formation during embryonic and fetal development. These represent the most critical periods in the span of life, beginning with the single tiny egg cell magically transformed by its encounter with an even smaller messenger carrying both the past and the future. Just as many aspects of life have their origins within this early period, so too does our understanding of the origins of cancer.

The Origins of Life

Life begins when a sperm fertilizes an egg. Immediately thereafter, the embryo rapidly expands from the solitary egg to a mass of cells that provides the building blocks to form each of the systems and organs of the body. The only requirement at this early stage of embryonic development is the generation of a sufficient population of cells. It's as if logs were being unloaded at a building site. At this stage, the logs are uncut on the lot and serve no special function other than waiting to be sawn and nailed somewhere in a yet-to-be-built house. Likewise at this point these early cells have no specialized function but retain the rudimentary capability to become any of the specialized cells of the more advanced fetus. Such a cell can become part of a liver system, or a lung—just as logs can be sawn to become part of a wall or a window ledge. Embryonic cells that have this power are called, appropriately, *totipotent* (pronounced *"toe-tee-PO-tent"*)—suggesting that they are "totally potent." These totipotent cells neither have, nor perform, any function other than to duplicate, over and over again, until a sufficient mass of cells has been generated. Once this critical mass of cellular building blocks has been generated, the genetic program—almost like a hidden system file in a computer—sends a message to end this rapid cellular proliferation. That's when cells begin

❖ Inspiration Point

Imagine if a person could somehow slice a fish in two, to create not two halves of one fish, but two identical-twin fish. That would be a messiah-like miracle, of course. But such miracles occur routinely at the cellular level.

to specialize and eventually form organs, tissue, and bodily systems. Because its function is to copy itself, a totipotent's "life" or *cell cycle* is extremely short, unlike *specialized* cells—ones with distinct functions already committed to being part of a more advanced fetus. A specialized cell has a prolonged cycle, spending most of its time functioning as part of an organ or bodily system. These organs and systems owe their creation to the embryonic totipotent cell.

When the totipotent cell is active, the cell cycle is unchecked. This occurs during the first two weeks of human embryonic development. Cells keep reproducing to make *mass*. One of the beauties of biology is a sophisticated molecular regulatory process. In a healthy embryo, this process determines when the unchecked cell cycle should be turned off. Thankfully so. If the unchecked cycles of cellular proliferation were to continue for the remainder of the nine months of gestation, the size of the infant at birth would approach the mass of the *moon*. This dramatic image is meant to focus your attention on the incredible procreation of an uncontrolled cellular cycle. In reality, life's elegant system that regulates the cell cycle is but a

❖ Inspiration Point

Learning scientific terms is a matter of principle. Most people would not buy a car without first learning about a car's miles per gallon rating, safety features, reliability record and other relevant information. Aren't you as vital as the vehicles you purchase? Isn't your body a vehicle for your soul or, if you're not religious, for your *mind*?

thin line between the exquisite life forms that make up our world and great blobs of simmering protoplasm. But how is this all related to cancer? The answer is simple: Cancer is a disease of the *cell cycle*. Cancer results when the body loses some of its control on cellular proliferation. In many ways, cancer is a reversion to those first two weeks of embryonic gestation when cells simply expand and divide to double their number in an unending continuum.

Normal cells remain in a kind of quiescence, or static state, for varying periods during which they carry out their intended functions. A liver cell, for instance, contributes to the liver system. A brain cell contributes to that organ. And so on. Then, they duplicate their chromosomes—replicating their genetic material—and begin to divide, creating two cells from one. Take a second to envision that. Imagine if a person could somehow slice a fish in two, to create not two halves of one fish but two identical-twin fish. That would be a messiah-like miracle, of course. But such miracles occur routinely at the cellular level. This process of replication and cell division is carried out by a subgroup of components—*action proteins*—which operate like engines within the cell.

❧ ❧ ❧

The Machinery of Life

"Machinery" is important to understanding both the life process . . . and cancer. Think of a large saw at a mill where a magic log, when cut in half, becomes two identical logs. The saw is the machinery (action proteins), and the magic log is the cell that replicates itself. You don't need to study the blueprint of that saw—how the various gears, screws and engine components turn the saw blade; you just need to know how the saw functions, splitting that magic log into two. You also need to know where the "off" switch is, to shut down the saw, or else your whole mill will fill up and overflow with identical logs. Likewise you don't need to know how the action proteins trigger replication and cell division; you just need to know that in normal cells, there is an off switch, too.

We realize it may take a little while to become familiar with the scientific terms that will be used in this chapter and throughout *Living Without Fear*. These are terms your doctor might use. But you might think, "As long as the doctor knows them, why should I?" Well, most people wouldn't dream of purchasing a car without first learning about the car's gas mileage rating, safety features, reliability record and other information found in the manual in the glove compartment. Aren't you as important as the vehicles you buy? Isn't your body a vehicle for your soul or, if you're not religious, for your *mind*? A popular women's hair-dye commercial says the product costs more but "you're worth it." Isn't your health or the health of your loved one worth the effort now, this day, at this moment? *Sure it is. So, take your time learning the terms for the various proteins that cause and cure cancer.* If you forget them in this or in later chapters, consult the glossary at the back of the book the same way that you would consult the car manual in your glove compartment when you need information about your car. To make your job easier, we have created metaphors to help you envision these essential, life-giving proteins.

So let's return, then, back to that "off" switch. The first thing to acknowledge is that "machine" proteins—the ones that govern cell replication—exist in two states: *active* and *inactive*. They're turned on and off by a *second* subgroup of protein molecules that remain dormant until they are chemically activated. How does *that* occur at this wondrous molecular level? Yet another protein, called "kinase" (pronounced *"KAI-nace"*) initiates a chemical reaction by adding a phosphate element to amino acids. That may sound complex, but it is really a simple but powerful chemical modification. It's as if this particular protein is a "mechanic" carrying a WD-40 spray can, only instead of lubricant, this can contains special phosphates. The mechanic—we'll call him, appropriately, *Kinase*—sallies to the "machine" protein and releases a chemical stream. In biology, this is called *phosphorylating* (spraying phosphates). The chemical causes a series of changes in the conformation of the complex protein molecule—the one that acts as the machine—almost as if it has been lubricated enough to "turn on." Things begin to hum. That machine molecule changes texture and position, allowing for *combined action*. In other words, it gets a piston-like boost. So activated, the "machine" proteins regulate replication and cell division, doing their work to complete the cycle.

Mechanics and Messengers

Back to those miniscule mechanics called *kinases.* When you encounter that scientific term, think of its root syllable—*kin*—as you would a last name. Just like people, many such kinases that influence or regulate the cell cycle have a "first" and "middle" name: *cyclin dependent kinases* or, abbreviated, *CDKs.* The CDKs are so called because they cannot do their job—spray their all-important phosphates on "machine" proteins—without help from yet another protein called cyclins (pronounced *"SIGH-klins"*). Put simply, those CDKs also need a boost so they can form a partnership with cyclins.

Enter now another group of central performers in this intricately automated morality play of cell-cycle regulation. These are "messenger" molecules known as E2F proteins. Think of these not as mechanics, but as letter-carriers that have one essential duty: delivering messages to activate genes that direct the production of the "machine" proteins that replicate cells. In a word, these E2F proteins deliver a letter read by genetic material, explaining how many machine proteins are needed to make enough cells for a system or tissue of the body.

Biologically speaking, all this is (or should be) rather routine. The process of producing machine proteins occurs via central mechanisms of molecular biology. Now *that's* a complex topic. But let's focus awhile on some basics which may be a bit cumbersome to comprehend at first. Let's begin then with "genes," those strands of long DNA molecules of the chromosomes. Genes communicate. They read bio-genetic information at the microscopic level, triggering production of specific protein molecules. While the E2F "messenger" proteins activate genes to make machine proteins needed to copy and divide cells, one group of proteins mentioned earlier—the cyclins—is vital in this process.

The CDKs, those spray-can mechanics, need a boost the way people do when they take vitamins, like a capsule of A or E. When people are inactive, they don't report to work. Same at the cellular level. The question is, just how do those CDKs bind and form a partnership with cyclins so they can do their jobs efficiently? For starters, imagine two brands of "cellular" vitamins in the mail bag of those letter-carrier E2F "messenger" proteins: *cyclin A* and *cyclin E*. The messengers deliver these "capsules" as if by address to specific kinase "mechanic" molecules known by a first name and a number; *cyclin dependent kinase 2* or *CDK2*.

Depending on which cyclin they have "ordered," these CDK2 mechanics go to work only after combining with cyclin A or cyclin E. As soon as they do, they get new names: E-CDK2, for one attaching to an E cyclin, and A-CDK2, for one attaching to an A cyclin. Because they have bonded, they are now known as complexes. Both complexes A-CDK2 and E-CDK2 can then phosphorylate, or spray their chemicals on, the action proteins and turn on the cell-cycle machinery to replicate cells. (**See Figure 1 to see the actual structure of CDK2.**)

Let's summarize to make this as clear as possible and realize that not long ago only the brightest molecular biologists understood these concepts. An E2F "messen-

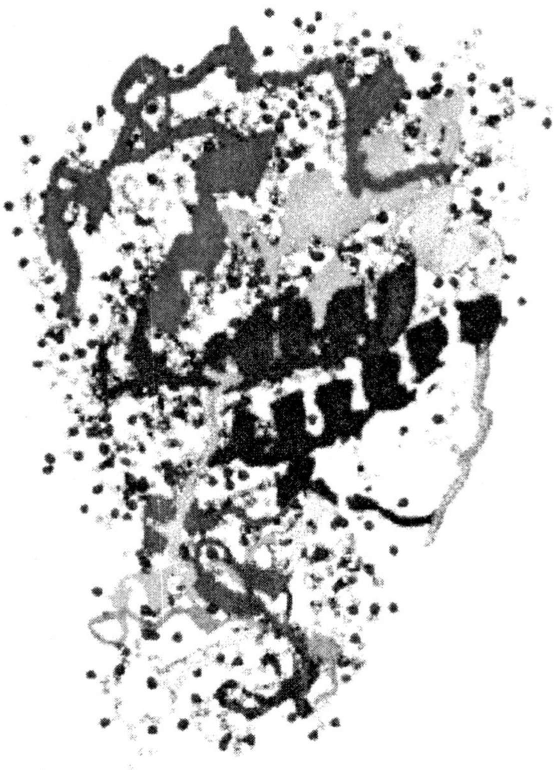

Figure 1.
Meet the "Mechanic" Protein

Seeing the actual structure of CDK2 enhances your molecular vision.

ger" protein triggers production of those "vitamin" cyclins A and E. Imagine a letter-carrier with samples of vitamins. The letter-carrier delivers those vitamins to the CDK2 "mechanics" reporting to work. Picture this: mechanics heading out to the mill where magical logs (cells) are produced. Those mechanics all have the same last name: Kinase. When they punch in, they are known as the *principal* kinases whose job is to activate machinery by spraying phosphates. The machinery produces identical cell upon cell that specialize by serving a bodily system, organ, or tissue. **(See Figures 2 and 3.)**

All this sounds terribly complex, but it isn't when you consider the miracle of the human body. In that context, this is but a relatively simple pathway that only represents the initial phases of cell-cycle regulation. "Regulation" is an apt term, too. This is all very fine-tuned. If E2F "messenger" proteins were always free to trigger production of action "mechanic" proteins, delivering cyclins to energize them, the cell cycle would continue unchecked in a horrible spate of runaway cell division. And, in a real sense, runaway cell division *is cancer*.

❧ ❧ ❧

The Origins of Cancer

In a healthy body, another protein prevents rampant cell division. It's a "guard" protein called retinoblastoma (pronounced *"re-tin-oh-blas-TOM-a"* and abbreviated *RB*). It firmly binds E2F and, in effect, halts letter-carriers on their delivery routes. In other words, no

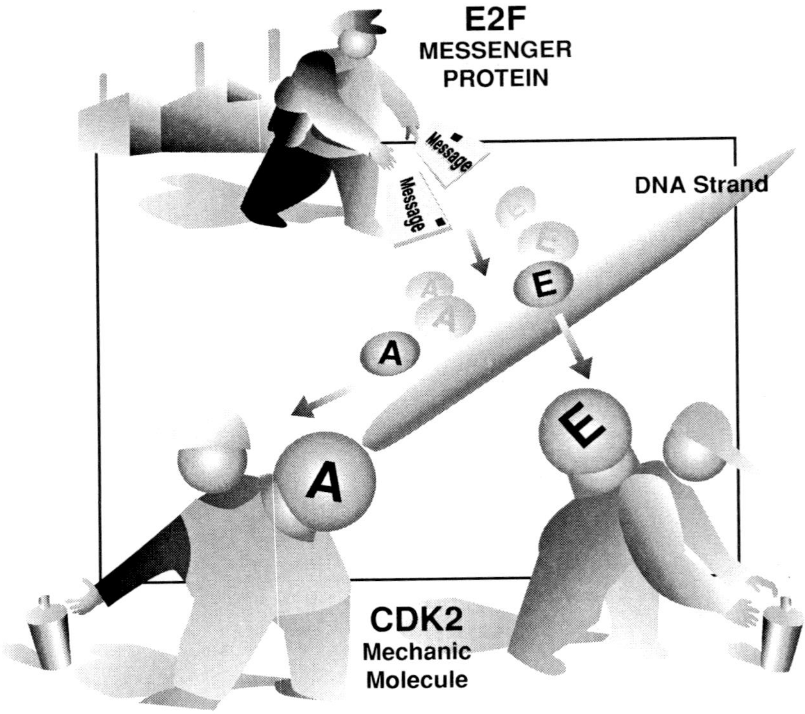

Figure 2.
The messenger protein E2F communicates with the DNA strand, and a "capsule" of cyclin A or E is sent to the CDK2 mechanic who then becomes known as A-CDK2 or E-CDK2, respectively.

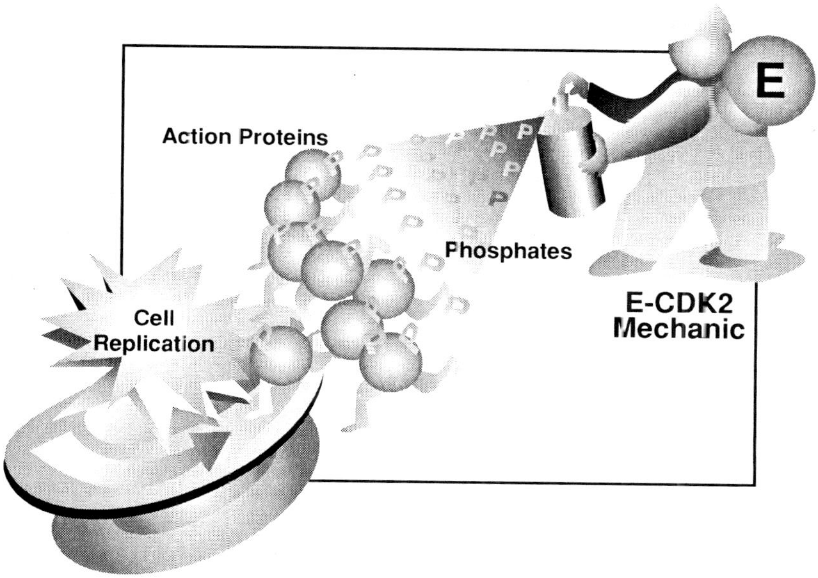

Figure 3.
The mechanic protein binds here with the capsule E, to become E-CDK2, and thus is able to phosphorylate, or spray phosphates on, the action proteins, resulting in a new copy of a cell.
(Note: The result is the same when CDK2 binds with the capsule A.)

messages are sent to the chromosomes of the cell to prompt the cell cycle. Thus, as long as all the E2F molecules of the cell are bound by RB molecules, which guard their unwarranted action, no cell replication can occur. **(See Figure 4.)**

The RB "guard" is an important protein both because of its role in cell-cycle regulation and because of its relevance to cancer. This protein's name alone suggests its connection to cancer. RB was first discovered as a gene that was altered in patients with the form of cancer known as retinoblastoma, an inheritable tumor of the eye. It was one of the early oncogenes (pronounced *"ONG-ka-jens"*), or cancer-related genes, identified by researchers several decades ago. But certainly this gene did not survive through the eons of evolution, nor was it created for the purpose of causing cancer. Neither this gene nor any other gene has the function of causing cancer, but like most other oncogenes, it is central to cell-cycle regulation. But since the RB "guard" blocks the cell cycle, how can that cycle be restarted? The answer to this question begins our discussion of how the cell cycle is controlled.

Now enter another cast and crew. We have another "vitamin" capsule so powerful it is labeled the "driver," or *cyclin D*. This is one of four gatekeepers associated with the cell cycle, and perhaps the most important gatekeeper with respect to the onset of cancer, as we will learn in Chapter Three. Right now, though, you also need to meet another molecular character—a master mechanic at a different address—known as cyclin-dependent kinase 4, or *CDK4*. He has a spray can, too. When he takes

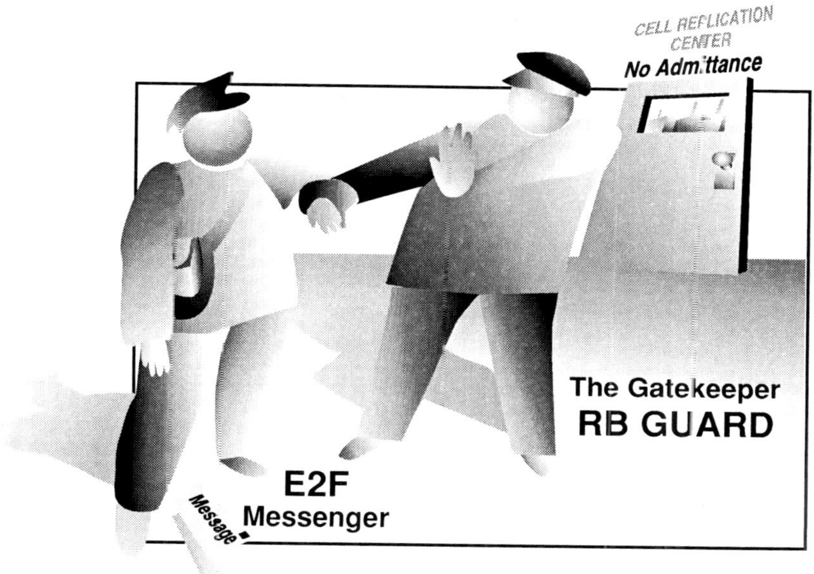

Figure 4.
One of the four gatekeepers known as the RB guard firmly binds the E2F messenger, preventing it from communicating with the DNA strand to send cyclins A or E to mechanic proteins, thereby shutting off cell replication.

"vitamin D," he sprays his phosphates not on the action "machine" protein but on the RB "guard." When the "guard" is phosphorylated it releases the "messenger" E2F, allowing it to signal the beginning of another cell cycle. **(See Figure 5.)**

All this is supervised by proteins that monitor or suppress this process. The cell cycle is controlled so that cell division is orchestrated precisely to maintain the cell number within an organ or tissue at a constant level. **(See Figures 6 and 7.)** These four gatekeepers of the cell cycle, two of which are often referred to by their atomic weights, are some of the most important molecules of life: the guard, the driver, the monitor (a *protein* with an atomic weight of *16000*, or *p16* for short), and the suppressor (a *protein* with an atomic weight of *53000*, or *p53)*. You already know the basic interaction between two of the gatekeepers—the guard and the driver. It is important to know as well that the monitor and the suppressor act in opposition to the driver to shut down the cell cycle. In Chapter Four, we'll explore the cancer process in detail. But at this point, note that the function of *three* of the four gatekeepers is to focus on that "off switch" to stop the cellular assembly line, flicked on by that all-powerful driver. Nonetheless, injury or damage to any gatekeeper has the same effect

> **❖ Inspiration Point**
>
> **The body is electric at the molecular level. But errors here can cause the cell cycle to go out of control, just as lives go out of control when you or loved ones hear the word "cancer." It's time to take back some of that control. If nothing else, you can achieve control over *fear*.**

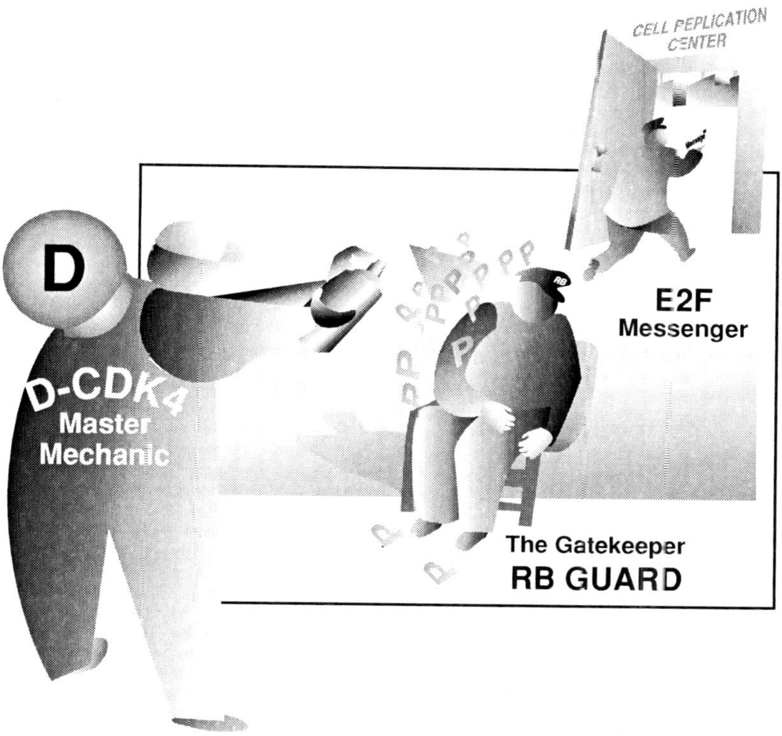

Figure 5.
The master mechanic D-CDK4 phosphorylates the RB guard, releasing the messenger and restarting the cell cycle shown in Figure 3.

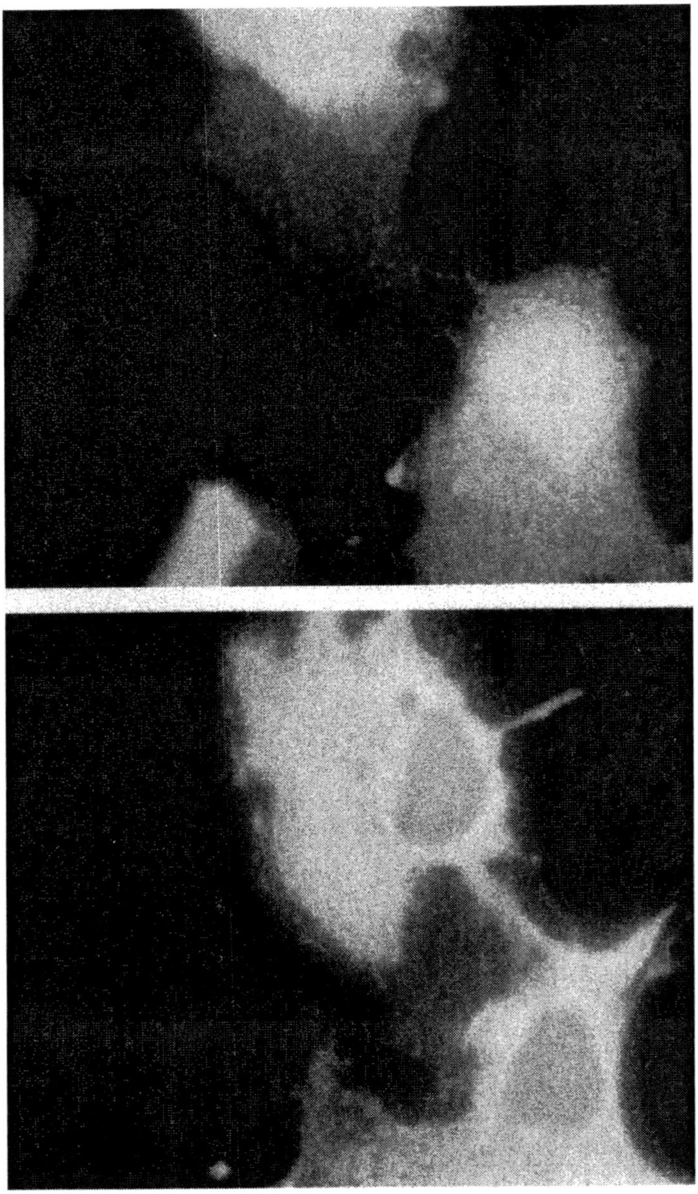

Figure 6.
Typical Normal Cells

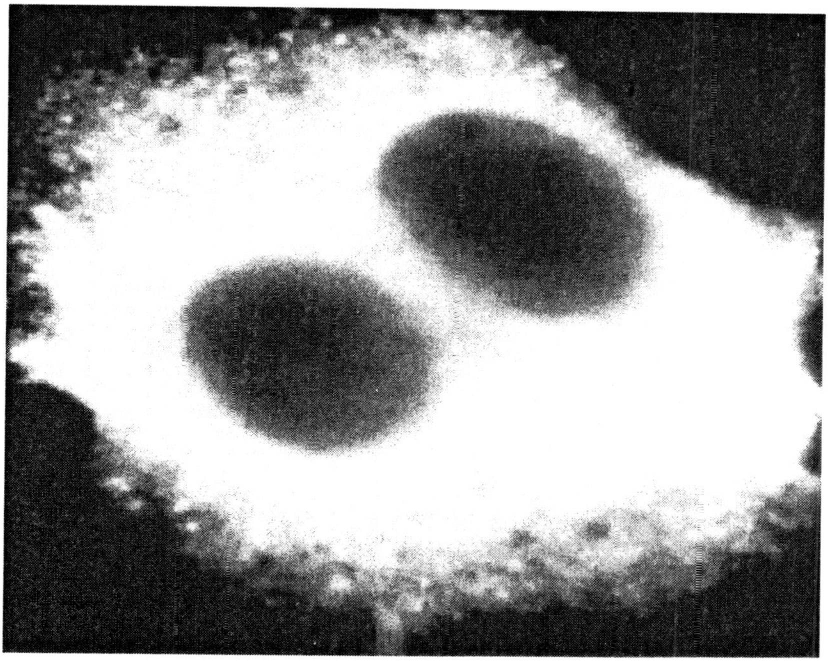

Figure 7.
A Cell Dividing

The Nucleus and the chromosomes inside have already duplicated and the cell is just about to divide into two.

upon the life process that the sudden collapse of a shift foreman would have on that assembly line.

The four gatekeepers monitor the system of cell-cycle control. But this is only half of the explanation of how the body maintains cellular *homeostasis,* or internal stability, within its organs. As you might anticipate, there is a darker side to the cell's life-span. Until a decade ago most medical scientists thought cell death was a random arbitrary phenomenon, but recently it has been shown that this view was incorrect. Just as the creation of cells is elegantly orchestrated, so also is their demise. Now scientists know that the death of cells is programmed, just as is the cell-replication process explained in this chapter. Although many cells of the body such as the muscle cells and some neuronal cells never divide and remain static throughout the life of the organism, dividing cells maintain their stability by controlled replication—producing a specific number of cells—and controlled *death.*

Keep in mind we're talking about *specialized* cells, ones with distinct functions, rather than *totipotent* cells. Specialized cells are born, or *generated,* from a population of seeding cells or stem cells in each tissue. Imagine orchards of beautiful but different varieties of trees—some that drop seed-cones, others that drop seed-propellers, and still others that drop seeds from flowers on limbs. Some of these trees don't even need to drop cones, propellers, or seeds. These varieties are like corkscrew willows and sprout offspring from shoots. Each of these orchards contains trees whose seeds or shoots make cells for some bodily organ, system, or tissue. In a real sense, the generation of specialized cells is similar to trees "dropping" seeds or sprouting "shoots." This happens when cells die. Each specialized cell goes through a certain number of divisions, usually 20 to 30, and then is programmed to perish. When cells perish, reaching their pre-determined life-span, a vital new cell is "born" again from the tissue's stem cell population, and the cycle is repeated. Less is known about the detailed mechanisms of programmed cell death than is now known about control of the cell cycle. But it's a fact that failure of the death program in cancer cells is as much a part of the *beginning* and *persistence* of a tumor as are errors in cell-cycle regulation explained earlier.

❧ ❧ ❧

Taking Control of the Process

Now you know the basics of the life and cancer origin. Simply explained, you contract cancer because of errors in cell-cycle regulation. To envision those errors, you have to understand key components explained here—the machine proteins, the messenger ones, the various CDKs and cyclins and, finally, the four gatekeepers. The body is electric at this level. But so are the consequences of cellular errors, causing havoc on the molecular assembly line, as if a factory foreman has collapsed, allowing the line to go out of control, just as lives go out of control when you or loved ones hear the word "cancer."

It's time to take back some of that control. If nothing else, you can achieve control over *fear*. And the best way to do that, as the great French paleontologist-philosopher Pierre Teilhard de Chardin maintained, *is to believe that you can.*

❦ ❦ ❦

Envisioning Exercise

Creative Visualization

Objective: To more fully understand what is happening in your body by visualizing events in your favor at the molecular and genetic level. To familiarize yourself with the various "characters" discussed: the messengers, mechanics and four gatekeepers—the guard, the driver, the monitor, and the suppressor.

1. Read through the chapter again to fully familiarize yourself with the concepts and "characters" discussed.

2. Then, begin to visualize a story taking place involving these characters. This story takes place within your body at the molecular and genetic level. In the story, events are happening in your favor. For example, if one of the gatekeeper "foremen" has collapsed—and the "assembly line" is about to spin out of control—perhaps one of the other three gatekeepers comes to the rescue to slow the assembly line until the guard revives enough to continue his job.

3. In your mind, flush out the plot of the story. Make it a positive one. Remember, during this exercise you are in complete control. Create the happy plot of a healing, healthy body.

4. Write down your story in a journal—just a few pages or more will do. If you are visually inclined, take a sketch pad and draw the characters in your story as well. Illustrating your story, even in a rudimentary way, helps you to understand what is happening at the molecular level in your body and envision success.

5. As an alternative (or an addition) to Step 4, describe your story into a tape recorder. Or, work on it with a friend or loved one and ask them to write and/or illustrate your story for you.

6. Contemplate and reflect on your positive story. This exercise should not only help you feel better, but also help you understand the processes at work in your own body. *This will enable you to experience less fear of cancer.*

Chapter Three

Mutants and Gatekeepers

The further the spiritual evolution of mankind advances, the more certain it seems to me that the path to genuine religiosity does not lie through the fear of life, and the fear of death, and blind faith, but through striving after rational knowledge.

—Albert Einstein 1879-1955

❧ ❧ ❧

You hear "mutation" or "mutant" so often watching television and movies that you may think these scientific terms are widely understood. Even Saturday morning cartoons have been filled with the likes of "Teenage Mutant Ninja Turtles," "X-Men" and other mutant characters that kids love. However, few people understand the meaning of mutation. To know it, you have to grasp the mechanisms that:

> **❖ Inspiration Point**
>
> **Humans stand out in creation and can be set apart from all other species—not at the DNA level, for we are made of the same stuff as animals—but at the consciousness level: *we can make what we envision.***

- ❖ Store and pass on genetic information—the blueprints of life—from generation to generation.
- ❖ Transcribe and translate that information into protein molecules.
- ❖ Govern those proteins from which the structures of our bodies are built and by which the functions of our bodies are performed.

Let's focus, for a moment, on the human body. To appreciate it, you first have to value the diversity of life, from the tiniest desert-dwelling microbes to the largest ocean-going mammal, whales. A few biologists have argued that the beaver, with its propensity to build, is the most spectacular creation, because its intelligence is based on design and architecture rather than hunting and killing. As such, the beaver is rather special in that most animals that develop intelligence are, or start out as, predators. Hunting requires strategy involving mapping, stalking and, in the case of humans, weapon-making. The beaver simply builds, and it is magnificent for this reason.

However, the human being is special in Earth's autobiography, first and foremost because it selected the brain as its mode of survival and then developed sophisticated languages that indirectly enabled the species to make almost whatever it imagined, from wagon wheels to space ships, from Galileo lenses to Hubble lenses. Other species like dolphins and chimpanzees may have a rich mental and emotional life—maybe even language—along with consciousness. But they cannot make what they envision beyond the essentials for survival, and because of that, their vision and consciousness are less extraordinary than that of humans. Many geneticists believe that we possess the ability to clone ourselves in the near future, although that has ethical ramifications beyond the scope of this book. But the fact that we can *make* this happen if we want—that we can engineer not only tools and space craft but, essentially, *ourselves*—puts us in a category which, frankly, is a rung or two above the beaver. And as far as this book is concerned, humans stand out in creation and can be set apart from all other species in the animal world—not at the DNA level, for we are made of the same stuff as beavers, whales, and apes—but at the consciousness level: *we can make what we envision.*

❧ ❧ ❧

Envisioning DNA

We may not be able to make what we envision immediately, for the artist flew on the wings of Pegasus long before the Wright brothers did at Kitty Hawk. Likewise we may take centuries to fathom the placebo effect and hearken it fully to heal ourselves. But you get the idea and the message: you may not be able to make yourself well —or even prevent the onset of cancer—simply by envisioning wellness. Neither should you feel that you cannot achieve at least a measure of wellness in this manner, because no one understands or can gauge the effectiveness of imaging techniques, including meditation and prayer. Just know what you're up against in the battle to defeat cancer, a formidable foe. You can strike cancer a blow, not only by evoking the placebo effect, but by *eliminating fear through knowledge.*

> **❖ Inspiration Point**
>
> **If we are life's most magnificent creation biologically, then you, too, possess magnificent powers. One of them is to envision the inestimable gift of life at the molecular level, thereby lessening fear in the fight against cancer.**

Knowledge is power. If we are life's most magnificent creation biologically, then you, too, possess magnificent powers. One of them is to envision the inestimable gift of life at the molecular level. All the data to depict how magnificent you truly are is found not in skyscrapers or space craft but in the tiny nucleus of each human cell. There, in this tiny organelle, lie the thin strands of our chromosomes, each of which are made up of a single, tightly wound and folded molecule of DNA. If stretched out to its full length, this miraculous molecule is several millimeters . . . yet only 0.0000020 millimeters wide. That's way too small to see with your naked eye, of course. And yet you possess the ability to envision something that tiny.

Say you live two kilometers from the ocean and sunbathe there everyday in the summer. One day you find an oyster shell washed clean by the waves, except for one perfect sun-sparked grain of sand in the middle of the marble-colored inside shell. You want to take that shell home but forget it on the boardwalk, remembering precisely where you left the shell only after you open your front door. Your mind travels instantaneously over that distance back to the boardwalk to the bench where you put the shell down momentarily to tie your sneakers, and although it is evening now, you still "see" that sun-sparked sand-grain in the middle of the shell. In your mind, you envisioned a sand-grain although you were quite far from it. That's rather amazing, isn't it, when you contemplate the dynamics of imagination? Now imagine that you had a tape measure that could stretch two kilometers; for argument's sake, let's call that distance the *length of a DNA molecule.* You have just entered the molecular landscape at that magnification. Now focus on the width of the sand grain. It's a rough basis of comparison, but that sand grain—compared to the two kilometers' length of DNA—represents *the width of a molecule.* You were able to "see" the grain of sand because *your imagination is able to transcend time and space.* Keep this in mind as we journey down our genetic pathways, using what seem like impossibly small numbers, with several zeros behind the decimal point. As long as *you* are behind the decimal point, you can see the light-year dimensions of the universe or the molecular ones of the cell.

The pseudo-sciences of numerology and astrology assign you numbers, by which you are supposed to measure your life. You can measure your life by your Social Security number or your credit card number or your lottery number or any other kind of number you chose, but they all pale in comparison to a number all of us share: 46. This represents the number of fragile DNA molecular strands that literally define us and our offspring.

We usually think of our heritage in terms of words. A family album, say. Or maybe a Bible or some other sacred text. We're beginning, as a society, to think of information not only as text but also as bits on a computer chip. That's a more apt symbol when we ponder DNA, because like your desktop, life has its own databank. And later in this

❖ Inspiration Point

Nature's language is perfect, and you are—quite literally—her *Word*, based on all the genetic words she has spoken before and about you through time.

chapter, when we discuss how the human gene stores information, we will have to use the computer as a metaphor for DNA. There's no need to rush, after all. You've just entered the molecular landscape. For many people, books rather than microchips remain the most common symbol of information storage. So we'll use that symbol momentarily to describe how DNA warehouses the data of life.

Surprisingly to lay people, the DNA molecule is a polymer (pronounced *"POL-ee-mer"*). You may know that substance as polystyrene (used in the housing of your refrigerator, say) and as polyester. Polymers are also found in minerals like diamonds and quartz and in concrete, rubber, and plastics. But they are found, too, in the natural world, in proteins, for instance; so in some sense, we are as molecular as polystyrene and polyester . . . but hardly plastic or artificial. And again, this has to do with repeating strands of DNA, each only 0.0000020 millimeters wide, so small only a high-powered microscope or the imagination can view it.

❧ ❧ ❧

The Language of Life

Unlike other common polymers, human DNA has four different repeating *units*—keystones of genetic language—whose arrangement and sequence encode all of life's information. We'll discuss those units later. For right now, just recognize that is one big truckload of data. You know the heft of a volume of the *Encyclopedia*

Britannica? The type is small, about 8 points, called agate or "fine print." Let's make an analogy between a volume of the encyclopedia and one of the DNA molecules within one of our chromosomes. First, it would be necessary to carefully cut out each line of text from each page of the encyclopedia volume and glue those lines end to end to make a continuing line of type. It would also be necessary to remove each of the spaces from between the words, along with punctuation. However, note that doing this would make the text unreadable as follows:

> anyofaclassofnaturalorsyntheticsubstancescomposedofverylarge-moleculesthataremultiplesofsimplerchemicalunitscalled-monomers

The sentence above defines "polymer" from the *Encyclopedia Britannica*. Properly typed and punctuated, it reads: *any of a class of natural or synthetic substances composed of very large molecules that are multiples of simpler chemical units called monomers*. But you can see how difficult it would be to easily reconstruct that sentence from the original one above. And it is virtually impossible for anyone to reconstruct the *entire* volume of type stretched out as a one mile long unreadable line of data. Here's why: suppose you came across a passage like this, purposefully short to make an important point: stopthatdrink-ingthisinstantteaisbetterforyou. Does the sentence read: "Stop that drinking this instant! Tea is better for you" or "Stop that drinking. This instant tea is better for you"? Now suppose, for a moment, that this volume of the encyclopedia was not written in English but in a language whose words only contained *three* letters. Here's a sample of that language: theboysawthebadconrevthenewredcar. Or, "The boy saw the bad con rev the new red car." A continuous line like this might seem funny at first, but soon you will adjust to the language because each word contains three letters.

Read this passage and see for yourself:

theboysawthebadconrevthenewredcarthecopdid-toofortheboygotmenwhoownthecartheconranoff-sadthemensayheyyouandcrynabhimsichimnowthe-copletouthisdogbuttheconhidlowandwaswaytoosly-foranycopyetnotthedogwhobithim

With a little practice, you should be able to make out a crime story about a con man who gets bitten by a police dog. Just put a space after every three-letter word and, though punctuation may vary, the plot should not:

The boy saw the bad con rev the new red car. The cop did, too, for the boy got men who own the car. The con ran off sad. The men say—"Hey you!"—and cry, "Nab him! Sic him!" Now the cop let out his dog but the con hid low and was way too sly for any cop . . . yet not the dog who bit him.

You can see that even a Nobel-Prize winning author would have an impossible time composing a novel in English using only three-letter words. Nature, though, is vastly more gifted than any prize-winning author on earth. Her language is perfect, and you are—quite literally—her *Word*, based on all the words she has spoken before and about you, from your father and your mother, to their parents and their parents, and so on until all individual family trees converge into one common homosapien orchard . . . or from one common homosapien set of parents. Some biologists and zoologists estimate that all human genes ever analyzed are more than 90% identical *in every person*. Which means the stranger seated across from you on the city bus is largely identical to you biologically. Same goes for any person on any bus in England, Japan, Australia, Vietnam, Kenya, Peru, China, or the United States. This kind of genetic uniformity is due, in part, to the DNA's uniform language.

This language not only can explain cancer but also offer hope for a cure. Here's why. Geneticists know the language of life and therefore can "read" the human genome (pronounced *"GEE-nome"*)—all the inheritable traits of a living creature. They are learning to read the genome as readily as you may have read the three-letter short story about the police dog above and spot any molecular misspellings—just as you are able to spot a four-letter word in the police-dog story. Go ahead and find the error:

The boy saw the bad con rev the new red car. The cop did, too, for the boy got men who own the car. The con ran off sad. The men say—"Hey you!"—and cry, "Nab him! Sic him!" Now the cop let out his dog but the con hid low and was way too sly for any cop . . . yet not the dog that bit him.

> **❖ Inspiration Point**
>
> **The genetic code is universal because it speaks on behalf of every person of every culture in every continent, peninsula, and island on earth and, for all we know, on other life-bearing planets elsewhere in the galaxy.**

In some sense, this is how a geneticist feels spotting a problem at the molecular level—in this case, the word "that" which contains four instead of three letters in this uniform language. But even the police-dog story does not do justice to the uniformity and precision of the genetic language that encodes all of its information into words of exactly three letters. To appreciate such precision, remember that genetic letters are encoded—or converted to language—by those four different repeating units in the polymeric structure of DNA.

This sounds rather technical. But the grammar of any language is technical at first, until you come to know it. So think of the polymeric structure of DNA as grammar. However, instead of letters, you'll use a little basic math. Since each word of the genetic tongue must be three units long, and since DNA has four distinct units with which to encode information, therefore only 4^3 or 64 combinations of words are possible. As far as languages go, this one is as miraculous as the totipotent cell that you read about in the second chapter. Your body requires this caliber of language because it articulates the "truth" of past, present, and future. And because your genome speaks the truth, and only that, it doesn't require a large vocabulary to persuade, argue, or refute. Likewise there are no Towers of Babble in the laboratories of science. The genetic code is universal because it speaks on behalf of every person of every culture in every continent, peninsula, and island on earth. No saint, seer, or messiah can use language as concisely. And it's important for you to respect this fact because, when you finish reading this book, you'll possess a basic genetic vocabulary and will experience what geneticists do on a daily basis, deciphering DNA's awesome scripture.

Consider this: The short story on the previous page about the police dog contains 68 total words and 43 different words. As already mentioned, the genetic language allows only 64 possible combinations and requires only 20 words to articulate creation. We need to focus some more on the English language to grasp the next revelation about the genetic code. The possible combinations in the police-dog story actually number in the hundreds because English, even at this rudimentary level, is imprecise. For instance, here is but one other version out of many that we can make out of the original story, again using 68 total words and the same 43 different ones:

> *Now the men say "hey" and let the sly con rev his red car. The new cop got low and hid; yet the bad men who own the dog saw him. The men cry out—"Sic him, boy! You nab the cop!"—but the cop ran off. The dog ran off, too, the way the men did. And the con was not any bit sad for the cop.*

Ponder, for a moment, how versatile English really is. We essentially made an opposite story of the exact same length using all the same words as in the original version. Such linguistic versatility is due to human consciousness empowered by imagination, and in its own way, is rich, rejuvenating, and rewarding. You're going to need that versatility, enrichment, and rejuvenation—not only to understand cancer, its treatment and prevention—but also to appreciate the conciseness of the genetic code. Unlike the language of DNA, English words bind easily to each other in an array of potential combinations. Consider the phrase "way too sly for any cop" in the first version of the police-dog story and "any bit sad" in the second. Can you see how individual words change meaning depending on how they are used? For example, the word "for" is used as a preposition and as a conjunction meaning "because." And the word "bit" is what the dog did to the con in the first story and how the con felt in the second!

DNA doesn't need to be so clever. It needs to be precise, for an important reason. The material needed to build a human body is made by proteins (or by other molecules that proteins manufacture themselves). So the DNA molecule only needs to speak "sentences" that describe each of the body's proteins. That's why the genetic code has a vocabulary of 20 words. Proteins are polymers of amino acids (pronounced *"a-MEAN-oh"*), a kind of acidic life-bestowing "alphabet soup," and since there are but 20 amino acids, life's language needs only 20 words . . . each encoding a specific amino acid.

In this sense, the genetic code resembles the English language. English, unlike many other languages, is positional. The meaning of a word depends on where you place a word in a sentence. Let's return to that earlier sentence: "Stop that drinking this instant! Tea is better for you." Switch the words around and see what you come up with. Here are a few of many possible variations:

1. Stop drinking this instant! That tea is better for you.
2. Stop that. Drinking this instant tea is better for you.

3. You stop that, for drinking this instant tea is better.
4. You better stop this drinking, for that is instant tea.
5. Stop that. Drinking this instant tea is better for you.
6. Stop that drinking. This instant tea is better for you.
7. Better stop that drinking. This instant tea is for you.
8. Stop drinking that. This better instant tea is for you.
9. Stop drinking that this instant. Tea is better for you.
10. Stop that instant-tea drinking. This is better for you.

Similarly, the order of the 20 "words" within the DNA strand determines the order of the amino acids within the protein. And when biological "words" are placed in a specific order, life has spoken a sentence that fully describes proteins within the molecular structure. But wait. There are as many as 33,000 different proteins within our bodies—roughly about a 5 percent of words found in an unabridged English dictionary. And yes, the genetic code can "speak" to, or align, the amino acids of each protein—essentially writing 33,000 different short stories using only 20 words in a maximum 64 different combinations. But how much molecular space does all this take? The fact is, DNA is not only miraculously concise and efficient, it also has space as vast as the two kilometers from house to beach described earlier in this chapter.

❧ ❧ ❧

The Warehouse of Life

Let's use a computer metaphor now, because we need to speak a little more precisely about data storage. Say you just bought a very modest desktop model with a 3.3 gigabyte hard drive, loaded only with Microsoft Windows. This is a special bio-computer, though, with unique functions. As easily as you load programs from a floppy or ZIP disk, you're going to load 33,000 proteins into the hard drive of your desktop. For starters, each of the 33,000 proteins—made up of amino acids in a particular order—has an average "length," or program size, of several hundred such acids. The good news is all 33,000 proteins can be stored on one ZIP disk because the program size for all such proteins measures between 30- and 50-megabytes. We'll use those numbers because all these proteins require about 30- to 50-million aligned units of the DNA polymer. For comparison, let's say that 1 byte of file space in this bio-computer equals 1 genetic unit. A ZIP disk contains at least 100 megabytes. Your unique computer can store the proteins with no problem. Information about each protein required to build the human body is easily encoded because the total length—or hard-drive space—of DNA within our chromosomes is more than *300* times as great. What on earth is all this extra DNA for?

> **❖ Inspiration Point**
>
> **We are awesome beings because genetic language orchestrates our protein molecules. Some of us have blue eyes; yet we don't have blue ears or blue toes!**

If we each simply produced all of our body's proteins continuously, at the same level, and in all the tissues of our body, we would not be the magnificent creatures we are, but only portions of a slimy sea of polymeric ooze. We are awesome beings because of the genetic language of our DNA and how it orchestrates, or expresses, each of our protein molecules. Some of us have blue eyes; yet we don't have blue ears or blue toes! Eyes are blue (or green or brown or hazel or some other hue) because of the expression of the eye pigment protein in a special group of cells within the eye. The blue-eye pigment gene is turned on there. Moreover, the gene for the person's blue pigment protein is in every cell of the body. And though these proteins are incredibly microscopic, we are sensitive to them. Our bodies are conscious of them.

Any pregnant woman knows that during her term she was a somewhat different person with different feelings and slightly different physiology. This feeling is based on fact. During pregnancy, hundreds of different proteins are being produced that are not otherwise present within the woman's body. But you don't have to be pregnant to sense the impact of proteins. When a person eats a sufficient amount of carbohydrates—a couple large powdered donuts, say—the body stops producing action proteins that normally make sugars out of body stores. The body doesn't require the sugars, because of the intake of carbohydrates; so the action proteins reproduce again only *after* our blood sugar level drops below normal. This is why a person who eats donuts for breakfast feels sluggish at about 10:30 in the morning. The lack of "action proteins" can make us, well, *inactive*! The phrase—"your body is sending you a message"—is factual genetically. It is useful to remember this because doing so demystifies DNA, and by demystifying it—imagining it as easily as you do a donut or a computer—you will envision more clearly the molecular landscape where life and cancer originate.

You probably can tell by now that our intent here not only is to describe the genetic language but also mutations, or errors, in its grammar or expression. We'll get there slowly, the way we did in the second chapter, describing how the various proteins interact with each other and how cancer occurs when one of the gatekeepers, for instance, collapses on the assembly line. Presently, we're still dealing with the hard-drive space of DNA. We already mentioned that one of the functions of a gene is to encode information to make a certain protein. But much of the rest of the DNA is there to control *when* and *where* this information is expressed. A gene truly has two functions and two parts. One function is information storage—a computer file containing bits of information; that part of the gene is called the *structural* portion. The other function is to restrict the reading and expression of that information, directing it only to the correct cell group and to the correct time or times required to access the data. The part of the gene that carries out this second function is called the *regulatory portion* (or "promoter") and is also responsible for determining how *much* of the protein is produced. This second part of a gene is much more complex and perhaps more important than the informational part. Consider it the "executive" file that launches a software program, for instance, determining when and where specific files go in correct directories in your computer.

❧ ❧ ❧

Mutants and Messengers

Remember the important "messenger" proteins, the E2Fs, that are central to cell-cycle regulation? In the second chapter we compared them to letter-carriers that have one essential duty: delivering messages to activate genes that direct production of the "machine" proteins, which replicate cells. The E2F proteins deliver letters, explaining how many machine proteins are needed to make enough cells for a system or tissue of the body. The messenger proteins do this by binding to the regulatory parts of genes. When a messenger does so, targeting a gene, it causes the twisted helix shape of the DNA of that gene to *untwist* slightly. It's as if the gene is opening a letter. When the DNA untwists, the information within the gene can be read, and the gene "turns on."

Those E2F messenger proteins have a special chemical structure. It allows them to recognize the unique sequence of "letter" units in the regulatory region of genes they want to turn on, as if they truly were letter-carriers who could recognize street numbers, to deliver mail. You might want to envision a molecular street now, winding around genes like houses separated by huge lots. By envisioning such a street, you will realize that much of the length of your DNA is not used as a blueprint to make proteins, but to generate (or house) unique targets (or addresses) for those messenger proteins. Only these letter-carriers do not normally deliver junk mail. Every "envelope" contains a telegram whose information maintains the cellular neighborhood. Should the messenger proteins deliver junk mail, information disrupting either the structural or regulatory portions of the gene, the houses in that neighborhood may collapse as if struck by a twister. *Damage to the molecular neighborhood is, in fact, a mutation.*

Let's use another metaphor to help make clear just how important these E2F-like "messenger" proteins are. A symphony conductor sends messages to musicians and, as such, is the central figure during a performance. The role of the messenger protein to targeted genes is as important to the life process as is the conductor to the creation of beautiful music. Simply by waving his or her baton, a conductor can evoke the tremolo of strings or the crash of a cymbal at precisely the right moment. Each action of the conductor on stage is purposeful; if he or she simply waved the baton as if swatting a fly, the orchestra would lapse into cacophony—the squeal of clarinets, the twang of violins, the boom of untimed timpani—making a mockery of the scripted music. Likewise, genes being randomly or continuously expressed would generate a hideous cacophony of proteins. Therefore, life commits much of its precious genetic material to orchestrating or conducting protein "musicians." In life's performance, the structural portions of genes must act in concert with the regulatory regions. Disruptions in either portion of a gene, especially involving the encoding of information, can have colossal effects on the life process resulting in serious ramifications leading to cancer.

❧ ❧ ❧

Implications of Molecular Errors

Simply defined, a genetic mutation is *any molecular change in either portion of a gene.* Typically this is sparked by a chemical reaction causing physical damage to any of the units of the DNA polymer serving as "letters" of the genetic language. In other words, a mutation is an error. Letters that make up molecular words become as unreadable as computer jargon. A mutation can also be any rearrangement of the sequence of these "letters," comparable to a misspelling. But these kinds of mistakes can have serious implications, precisely because the genetic language is so compact, concise and efficient. The very means by which DNA encodes information makes it especially susceptible to mutation. Reaction with certain chemical substances can simply change one DNA unit or "letter" into another and cause the wrong animo acid to be placed at a certain position of the protein it encodes—just like words in an English sentence, placed in the wrong position, can change the entire meaning of that sentence. When that happens genetically, a vital protein can become non-functional, or other chemicals can simply delete one unit and therefore one letter from the message. Since the words within the genetic messages are not separated by spaces, the single deletion of one "letter" in any of these messages can turn the message into complete nonsense. For example, imagine the phrase "see the rat" made up of words of only three letters but strung together without spaces between the words so as to read "seetherat." Now imagine the removal of one letter "e" from "see" in the sentence. The meaning now becomes "setherat . . ." or "set her at. . . ." However, genetically, such mistakes rarely have any meaning because the sentences are longer and grouped in words of only three letters.

The genetic language is sensitive to chemicals, we said. More and more chemical substances in our environment are reacting with DNA and causing genetic mutations. The best known of these chemical agents are a group of molecules formed at the high temperatures of combustion in burning cigarettes. Smoke is inhaled into the lungs. The same type of mutation-causing chemicals are formed when fatty meats are cooked over open flames. These mutagens (pronounced *"MYOOT-a-jens"*) and their connection with cancer are generally well known; yet they are only a small number of the increasing number of mutagenic substances plaguing our environment. But even if all such agents could be kept away from our DNA molecules, natural events would continually introduce mutations into our genes. Sunlight causes a photochemical reaction within the DNA molecule that results in the random deletion of "letter" units from DNA messages. Chromosomes sometimes simply break into chromosomal fragments that fuse with other chromosomes to align the regulatory region of one gene with the structural region of another. That creates strange genetic mixtures, as surreal as a

> **❖ Inspiration Point**
>
> **"Mutation" is inevitable, an important part of the life process. Mutation generates the diversity from which successful life forms are selected. Knowing this, and more, you will be less apt to fear the word.**

Ferrari instead of a tractor pulling a manure spreader. Mutation is inevitable. Mutation is a part of life. Mutation generates the diversity from which successful life forms are selected. In other words, mutation keeps generating or evolving different creatures for different habitats on earth, in concert with changing environments or weather patterns or any number of natural, cosmic, and/or man-made phenomena. That's why some biologists feel that cloning animals or even humans one day—using genetic material from one point in time to create an animal or human in another—will result in inferior rather than superior beings, because the donor genes have not evolved sufficiently via mutation.

> **❖ Inspiration Point**
>
> **Four specific proteins are known as "gatekeepers" of the cell cycle. They regulate the life process and possess super-cellular powers. Knowing how they function demystifies cancer and empowers you with information, both of which should lessen fear.**

To grasp this, and make a point about mutation, let's imagine a science fiction scenario with an unhappy ending. It's the year 2079, and the depletion of the ozone is threatening humankind. By now, biologists can clone humans and, from a lock of his famous hair, they have access to Albert Einstein's genome. Of course the clone wouldn't *be* Einstein. Cloning is simply a remake of an older chassis like a model T automobile. The driver would not be Henry Ford, but some other soul behind the genetic wheel. Nonetheless, the clone of Einstein possesses a genius intellect and may help restore the ozone and earth's fate.

These 21st Century biologists believe that there is just enough time to clone, rear, and educate the Einstein clone to young adulthood so that he can use his intellect in combination with technological advances to resolve the urgent environmental problem. The clone is born and grows up unhealthy. The problem? Einstein was born in 1879, two centuries earlier. His clone's 19th Century genes have not evolved sufficiently to handle the increased levels of ultraviolet light on skin, resulting in early melanoma and premature death. The ozone problem worsens, and earth is doomed. Of course, this scenario would depend on particulars of the clone's genome and other factors; but the science fiction story above also demonstrates *why* mutation occurs in nature.

❧ ❧ ❧

Unnatural Born Mutants

While mutation may be natural, its frequency in an ideal environment should be low. Actually, mutation occurs within the cells of each of us. No one is free of mutagenic events within their DNA, but these mutations usually have no consequence. For example, the structural gene that encodes the pigment protein of the eye exists in all cells. So a mutation there can take place in any cell—*except pigmented ones of the eye*—without effect. That's because this particular gene is not expressed anywhere else. That's why blue-eyed people don't have blue ears or toes. Even a mutation in a gene that is expressed within the cell where the mutation occurs—the pigmented one of the eye, say—has little consequence since the abnormal cell is only one of *billions* of cells within its tissue. So one cell not performing its function makes no difference. The good news is that almost *no* mutations within any *cells*, except sperm and egg cells, have any negative consequences. The bad news is that mutations in the *genes* regulating the cell cycle can lead to cancer. In fact, mutations in the genes-coding for the four gatekeepers—the guard, the monitor, the suppressor, and the driver, described in Chapter Two—can have significant consequences. Why do these mutations differ so dramatically from others?

The gatekeepers are impressive because they regulate the life process. In some sense, they are superheroes with special powers. An eye cell is an eye cell, one out of billions, but a eye cell containing a mutant gatekeeper gene has a dramatic advantage over its billions of neighbors. In a word, it can disrupt the cell cycle, causing cell division and proliferation at an alarming rate. Cells of the mutant are mutants as well. They can divide so much faster than other cells of the tissue that the cellular neighborhood goes bad, populated by arch-enemies who—unlike normal cells of a tissue or organ—will not contribute to that system but rob it, literally, of nutrients and possessions and, ultimately, life. Mutations in the four gatekeeper genes are associated with most cancers, but the nature of these mutations is different and diverse.

You remember the powerful "driver," or cyclin D, from the second chapter? That's the gatekeeper capsule that bonds with CDK4, which sprays phosphates on the gatekeeper "guard." When that happens, the guard releases the "messenger" E2F, allowing it to signal the beginning of another cell cycle. Cyclin D is over-expressed, or present in overabundance, in many human cancers, caused by an array of mutations. Some of these mutations change the sequence of "letter" units within the regulatory region of the driver gene, allowing letter-carriers to turn it on or allow it to remain on longer, thereby producing more and more "driver" proteins.

Other "driver" gene mutations are the result of chromosomal breakage. When the fragments re-connect in the wrong sequence, they cause the regulatory region of one gene to attach to the structural region of another. The technical term for this phenomenon is "*chromosomal translocation*," and that can have dramatic effects when it involves the "driver" gene. Only very small amounts of the "driver" protein are needed to regulate normal cell cycling, so the regulatory region of that gene should produce only small amounts of this protein. That's why errant combinations of fragments can be deadly. Imagine the result if a regulatory region from a gene that produces large amounts of protein—a muscle gene, say—were aligned with the structural gene of the driver of the cell's cycle. The result would be a *huge* overprotection of the driver. In other words, more and more drivers would be produced and, consequently, mutant cells would be dividing and replicating at an extremely rapid rate.

Let's return to that earlier analogy used to illustrate the surreal combinations of chromosomal translocation: a Ferrari pulling a manure spreader. Spreading manure on crop fields is one of the least appealing chores of farm life. A manure spreader slowly moves its load into the beaters that fling it evenly onto the field. This is done by slowly moving slats beneath the load, connected by gears to wheels of the machine. As long as the tractor pulling the spreader moves at a steady slow rate, the process of distributing its load is efficient. But imagine a Ferrari instead of a tractor barreling down a drag strip at more than 100 mph and—you guessed it—not pulling a parachute, to slow its speed at the end of the race, but a manure spreader. The manure would not spread as much as *fly* in huge quantities on spectators along the strip. At the molecular level, that's the probable outcome of a chromosomal translocation associated with the cell cycle "driver" gene. And as you might anticipate, a significant percentage of lymphomas, adenomas, squamous cell carcinomas, esophageal carcinomas, bladder cancers, small-cell lung tumors and breast cancers and more have mutations in the regulatory region of the cell cycle "driver" gene, cyclin D. Many of these mutations are chromosomal translocations.

Only the "driver" acts to open the gate to cell division. As such, it is as much as gate*buster* as a gatekeeper. The other gatekeepers act in opposition to the "driver" to close down the cycle. But the driver isn't an arch-enemy. Neither is it a mutant. But when produced in overabundance, it can disturb normal cell cycling and that can lead to cancer. In fact, any mutation that either destroys or alters the delicate balance among the four gatekeepers—thereby allowing rapid cycling of a cell—triggers the onset of cancer. For example, mutations causing the gatekeeper guard to go defective have unfortunate effects upon cell-cycle regulation and are associated with several very aggressive cancers such as small-cell carcinomas of the lung as well as with retinoblastoma, with which the "driver" and RB guard are associated. But the most common targets of mutations are two other gatekeepers—p53, known as the "suppressor," and to a lesser extent p16, known as the "monitor." By far the "suppressor" gene is the most frequently mutated gene in human cancer and p16 is now being shown to be defective in an increasing number of tumors.

❧ ❧ ❧

Demystifying Cancer

Cancer typically defies generalizations. But generalizing is necessary now if we wish to envision events at the molecular level. A scientist or a physician reading this text would say that information presented in the first three chapters here, especially about the four gatekeepers, is basically correct but oversimplified. The scientist and physician would be right. More than 100 cancer-related genes have now been identified, and this number alone indicates that there are many more "actors" in the morality play of cancer than the four gatekeepers. Nonetheless, the gatekeepers are special because they provide a principal logic by which you can chart the molecular terrain. Most of the 100-plus "actors" in oncogenesis are genes converting genetic language that influences the four gatekeepers and triggers, through one process or another, mutants that spawn uncontrolled cell replication and division. As such, almost all cancers involve one of the four gatekeepers. Knowing how they should function, and why cancer can occur when they do not, empowers more than the imagination. It demystifies cancer, which only decades ago was seen as a social curse cast upon those afflicted as if by a mutant god hell-bent on human destruction. Yes, cancer can be that powerful. But as mentioned repeatedly here, knowledge is power, too, and essential in quelling fear.

❧ ❧ ❧

Courage, Fear and Hope

Ethicists often observe that there are two types of courage: physical and moral. As most combat veterans will tell you, physical courage is a matter of timing and control. Commandos with Type A personalities may be invincible warriors on the battlefield, as long as they are stalking the enemy. But even these commandos can be frightened into quick submission if ambushed at the precise moment, depriving them of timing and control. So physical courage, especially the type celebrated in action movies and sporting events, is of little use to you in the war against cancer, whose battle tactics deprive its prey of time and a sense of control.

Fear is an ethical construct, too. As history has shown, fear thrives in the *absence of fact,* as evidenced by the burning of scientists as heretics in medieval Europe and of women as witches in Salem, Massachusetts. Loss of control occurs when we cannot make sense of events or feel that they are beyond our comprehension. As if some tyrannical overlord from on high is punishing us or some evil arch-enemy from below is targeting us . . . all because of a long-forgotten misdeed or sin. When we feel that way, fear blossoms and is expressed as *guilt*. Fear is expressed as *anger* when we cannot forgive, because to forgive, you have to understand what you are forgiving and why. To know what to forgive, you contemplate facts, mulling them over until you grasp the reasons behind an action, situation, or event. Otherwise you stay angry and lapse at the slightest provocation into the bottomless underworld of fear. Finally, when fearful, your perception is skewed so that you cannot appreciate the blessings in your life. Your awareness dims along with your mind and creates an inner habitat of *hopelessness*. Cancer thrives in such an environment, as many nurses and physicians will attest, sensing who will survive in the ward—who has "the will to live"—and who lacks it, allowing fear to overcome the self or soul.

Moral courage rebuts fear. It is not based on timing and control but on will and awareness. By reading this book and envisioning events at the molecular level, we hope:

- To enhance your knowledge by understanding the basics of the genetic language. As a result, you may experience a lessening of fear.
- To demystify cancer by understanding mutation as an environmental outcome. As a result, you may experience a lessening of guilt.
- To explain mutagens as a natural phenomenon that makes earthly existence possible. As

a result, you may experience a sense of forgiveness.

- To envision all this imaginatively in a manner that bestows hope.

Envisioning Exercise

Focus on the Positive

Objective: To crowd out the fear and negative voices in your mind by focusing on positive aspects in your life.

Start a daily journal to celebrate the blessings in your life. Your focus will be on the part of the glass that is "half-full," not the part that is "half-empty." If you cannot physically do this, ask someone to take down your observations.

1. Begin by making a list of all things meaningful to you—these can be anything—from the breath that you take to the breeze that you feel, from the memory of love to the realization thereof. You celebrate your consciousness by naming your favorite animals, insects, trees, flowers, and other expressions of your immediate or remembered environments. Explore why these things are meaningful to you.

2. Then, focus on the people in your life who are supporting you with their actions and with their presence and positive energy. Write about their value to you. You may even choose to share your thoughts with them.

3. As you get involved with your journal, make an effort to write creatively—compose a poem or story.

Perhaps you can envision and write about those four gatekeepers—the driver, the guard, the monitor and the suppressor—as mythical beings working hard on your behalf. In a real sense they are your personal heroes, every bit as powerful as the archangels of paradise—Michael, Gabriel, Raphael, and Uriel—or the four Native American spirits—the great North, South, East and West winds. These molecular gatekeepers maintain your own inner Eden, however fallen.

Today, however, your inner garden is lush.

Chapter Four

The Twisted Path from Pre-Cancer to Cancer

There's another emotion associated with art, which is not of the beautiful but of the sublime. What we call monsters can be experienced as sublime. They represent powers too vast for the normal forms of life to contain them. An immense expanse of space is sublime. . . . For example, some of the temple gardens in Japan are designed so that you will first be experiencing close-in, intimate arrangements. Meanwhile, you're climbing, until suddenly you break past a screen and an expanse of horizon opens out, and . . . your consciousness expands to an experience of the sublime.

—Joseph Campbell (1904-1987)

The following is a recollection of co-author Michael Bugeja:

My earliest memory happened at age 5 outside my home in Lyndhurst, New Jersey, an enclave of New York City. The year was 1957, and I was standing curbside with my mother. I remember the blue Pontiac of my mother's brother approaching and then slowing to a stop. I could see my beloved grandfather on the passenger side. My grandfather, known affectionately as "Pop," immediately opened the door and stretched out his arms to receive me. I was excited. Whenever I saw Pop, it was a special occasion, because the bald-headed once-muscular man was the head of his ethnic family, and as such, commanded respect. And I was grandfather's favorite, a coveted honor.

In the 1920s Pop emigrated from Malta to America so that his family had a better chance of survival. A biologist might say that the grandfather's feelings for me had as much to do with Darwin's theory of evolution, applied culturally, as with familial love. After all, I was already seen as intelligent enough to solidify the family's foothold in the United States, the land of opportunity. In a quarter century's time, Pop was able to buy and eventually bequeath a home to my mother.

Darwinism, of course, has its down side. This carving out of new habitat took its toll on Pop, the head of the clan. As an immigrant, he could only find work as a laborer at the cork factories in nearby Newark, New Jersey. And although Pop's family would thrive, fulfilling the American dream, the patriarch would suffer personally and develop lung cancer from inhaling cork dust and toxic chemicals. His body could not tolerate the rapid change of environment. Accustomed to the then-pristine waters of the southern Mediterranean, Pop just couldn't adapt to the industrial pollution that accompanied prosperity in North America. And at age 63, he was dying.

Although my grandfather might have favored me for social reasons, I genuinely loved the older man because he lavished attention on me in an otherwise work-oriented ethnic family. But something was very wrong today at the curb. As I was about to leap into Pop's arms, my mother whisked me up in her arms and begged my grandfather not to touch me. She, too, was under the influence of biology and environment. She had lived in Malta until age 3, when her father had summoned her and her mother to America. She married in her 20s and quickly became pregnant, losing three babies to stillbirth and miscarriage before I was born—her only son. Nonetheless on that day, her behavior was suspect, even to me. Under normal circumstances, her actions would have constituted a scandalous betrayal; Pop, after all, was the patriarch and could inflict severe punishment—disowning her and writing her out of his will—for such an offense, the withholding of her son from his grandfather's embrace.

Suddenly, however, my grandfather appeared to have lost his powers. This was obvious to me, listening to him plead with my mother to hold her son "one last time." My mother clutched me and cried "no" in Maltese and turned away to walk back to the house. Pop, hobbled by cancer, could not get out of the car to follow. Finally he agreed and closed the passenger door of the Pontiac, vowing not to touch me. My mother turned around again and came closer to the curb, allowing the old man to whisper goodbye from a "safe" distance. And then Pop solemnly nodded to my uncle, who pulled away from the curb, driving my grandfather to the hospital, never to be seen again.

> **❖ Inspiration Point**
>
> **Cancer still strikes fear because few people understand what is occurring at the molecular level. Actually, genetic mutations that can lead to cancer occur routinely in our bodies. In early stages, healthy cells vastly outnumber mutations in the cellular neighborhood.**

This was an all-too-common scene in the 1950s, because of fear of cancer. Many people then falsely believed that cancer, like leprosy, was contagious and so forbade contact in the advanced stages, yet another indignity in a myriad of indignities associated with this disease.

In the decades to follow, lay people have learned much about cancer. The media, in particular, have dispelled myths like the one above and also have encouraged the medical community to share information with patients and their families. For instance, Michael Bugeja's grandfather knew that he was going to die—not because doctors informed him, typically withholding such information from terminal patients—but because his body communicated it to him. His *consciousness* knew it. Yet fear thrived throughout his illness because he and his relatives lacked knowledge.

The more people learn about cancer, the less they fear it. And while present-day information about symptoms of the disease, along with its possible triggers—smoking tobacco and eating fatty foods, for instance—are commonly known, cancer still strikes fear in families because few people understand what is occurring at the molecular level. If they did, they would realize that genetic mutations that can lead to cancer occur routinely in our bodies. After all, the four gatekeeper genes are ominous targets of mutations, as are at least 100 other potential cancer-initiating genes in each of our billions of cells. So the first step toward losing fear of cancer is to ask a courageous question: *Why doesn't the constant presence of mutational agents in our environment begin cancers in all of us?* The simple answer to this question is that it probably does.

Traveling the Cellular Landscape

Having read the first three chapters, you already know more than most people about the genetic causes of cancer. You realize, for instance, that a mutagenic "hit"—a chromosomal translocation in one of the many cancer-related genes—may cause a cell's cycle to spin out of control, especially if it involves one of the four gatekeepers. Suddenly the mutant cell's doubling rate dwarfs that of its neighbors; but in every other way, it is just like those neighbors and needs sustenance and a network of cellular associates to keep on doubling and thriving. More importantly, the mutant is not yet a cancer cell. True, one

❖ Inspiration Point

Most cells are good citizens and know the value of DNA, which promises miraculous abundance. To protect its precious neighborhood from damage, each cell carefully monitors how well its genetic message has been copied. In fact, cells are fanatic monitors of their own bloodlines.

day it might trigger cancer and change the fabric of the cellular neighborhood. But at this stage, the normal cells outnumber the mutants and contribute to the organ, tissue, or system associated with that neighborhood. So all is well. So well that if you were to travel the cellular landscape along the winding path of intestinal tissue, you would see an orderly city for miles and miles, with only occasional clusters of mutant cells and their decedents. Nonetheless, you'd notice them when you spotted them. How could you miss a column of Ferraris pulling manure spreaders on cropland or a flotilla of tug boats dragging missile launchers across Central Park? That's how obvious some mutant clusters look to geneticists. Such clusters have a name: hyperplasia (pronounced *"HIGH-per-PLAY-she-ah"*), otherwise known as a pre-cancerous tissue, or a non-malignant tumor. And yet these clusters are still a long, long way from becoming cancer. Drive long enough along the contour of any organ and you're apt to see sections of hyperplasia. The question before us in this chapter is how, exactly, does such a pre-cancerous cluster grow and eventually overtake the neighborhood, progressing to a full-blown cancer?

Back to those gatekeeper genes, so important to molecular health and well-being. As you know, the guard, the driver, the monitor, and the suppressor control the cell cycle. When mutations disturb it, there are two direct results. First, genetic replication spirals out of control, as you learned in the previous chapters. But of almost equal importance is the effect of these mutations on DNA repair, in many ways like street repair and home improvement in the molecular neighborhood.

Let's continue with that metaphor a while longer. Most cells are good citizens and know the value of DNA, which promises miraculous abundance. To protect its precious DNA from damage and mutation, each cell carefully monitors how well its genetic message has been copied following each cycle of DNA replication. In some sense, this is not far removed from Michael Bugeja's grandfather carefully monitoring how well his progeny would do in America in future generations of his bloodline. Cells are fanatic monitors of their own bloodlines. For instance, they often catch errors in the transcription of genetic information from the parent cell to one of its two daughter cells, following cell division. When this happens, the incorrect stretch of the daughter cell's DNA is removed and carefully replaced by the correct information. The cellular machinery is able to do this because DNA is composed of two strands twisted around each other. One of the strands comes directly from the parent cell unchanged and the other is a newly made strand. By comparing the two strands and looking for any differences, the cellular machinery can easily detect any errors in replication.

Like parents, cells spend much of their time between births of their offspring monitoring how well the "replication" went. Like parents, cells also spend much of their normal life cycles maintaining their habitat, in this case, devoting energy and resources to DNA repair. And just as it might happen to diseased parents who continually bear children with the same congenital illnesses, who in turn continually bear children—with little or no attention paid to maintaining their habitat—well, things break down . . . even as they amass. This is what happens to the DNA repair process when the span between cell cycles is dramatically decreased. Clearly, as the cell cycle spins out of control, DNA repair suffers since less time is available for upkeep, maintenance, and reconstruction. The repair is done by street crews—action proteins of DNA that slowly move up and down its long, twisted strands—much like tiny repavement trucks looking for and fixing potholes and road wear to streets in the cellular neighborhood. If the street crews don't have time to repair damage to the roadway, overpass, or bridge, cars traveling on that street will encounter disaster. It's as if a mother driving to the hospital to bear her next child spirals out of control after her car hits a large pothole. Likewise if the next cycle begins before the DNA repair machinery can correct a mistake from the previous replication cycle—fixing a figurative pothole, for instance—an otherwise temporary mistake becomes a permanent mutation in the cell's genetic heritage.

In real life, that pothole would be repaired so that other mothers driving to the hospital will not suffer a similar fate. But genetic mistakes like this are more dramatic, condemning every other mother traveling that stretch of DNA to spiral out of control at that juncture, as in the original "accident," or mutation. In other words, DNA repair is critical. The cell has one chance to patch common mistakes often made by the DNA replication machinery. It's as if the cell has a map to compare how the original route to the hospital should look and carefully studies the route the daughter will take, ordering repairs when it finds any discrepancies. Once a mistake has been missed and the daughter cell is replicated by its own offspring, the unrepaired stretch of its DNA strand now becomes the new *parental* strand. That means one of its daughters and the granddaughter of the original correct cell now contains a "parental" strand with the mistake embedded in it. Forever afterward this mistake or mutation will be carefully maintained by the same repair system that makes sure the new daughter strands exactly copy their parental strand. Now street crews get a mutant map that doesn't show a smooth path to the hospital but one that contains a road hazard. (A word about that "map." It's more like a mold than folded paper, because the left strand of DNA is a template for the right. In other words, both sides should be a perfect "fit." When they aren't, an error—in our metaphor, a "road hazard"—has been detected, and repair crews are dispatched.) But now, because of a defect in the map, repair crews do not fix the hazard because the map has a signpost that states: "Large Pot Hole Located Here." So car upon car containing pregnant "mother"-cells replicating too quickly pile up at the accident site, one after another, as found in hyperplasia. So not only does a mutagenic "hit" in one of the gatekeeper genes cause the resulting cell to loose control of its cycle, it also increases the future rate of mutation in this cell and all of its decedents. In addition, one of the gene groups often found mutated in cancer cells, probably because of this early faulty DNA repair, is that class of genes responsible for directing the production of the action proteins of DNA repair. Such a double mutant, with defective cell-cycle control and faulty DNA repair, can now accumulate mutations at an alarming rate. Tragically, it is exactly this accumulation of multiple mutations one after the other that causes pre-cancer to develop into cancer.

❧ ❧ ❧

The Cellular Road to Cancer

As we have noted from the start, cancer is not a disease but a class of diseases. That's why "secondary" mutations (genetic errors described in the paragraph above)—and the sequence in which they must occur to result in cancer—differs for each cell type and, therefore, for each cancer. It is possible to explain all of these scenarios, and how each leads to a different type of cancer; but doing so would expand this chapter to encyclopedia length. That analogy should give you an idea of the complexity of cancer confronting geneticists every day in the laboratory. You don't need to know all that. You need to know the process at the molecular level so that you envision how cancer develops, enhancing your consciousness so that you can muster it at the end of this chapter. That's why the process of a single cancer is presented here—a cancer for which the path from the initial mutational hit to the mature disease is now reasonably well understood.

Colorectal cancer is one of the most widespread of human cancers in the United States. The specialized cells of the colon's intestinal lining exist in an exceptional environment. For starters, these cells are actively involved in the absorption of nutrients from food passing along their path. The movement of food fibers exerts a physical force on these cells. Both of those elements—food absorption and passage—require a much higher turnover rate than found in most other cells. In other words, colon cells must replicate quicker because the wear-and-tear on them is greater than that of most other cells associated with different organs, systems, or tissues. So colon cells replicate dramatically faster than do other counterparts of the body, although the cycle is finely tuned by biological machinery at the molecular level. The machinery realizes that colon cells have shorter lifespans and so balances the replication of new cells with the destruction of old ones in the passing ebb and flow of the food-processing intestine and colon.

We've discussed how tissues maintain their constant cell number by controlling both the rate of cell cycling and the rate of programmed cell death. In an earlier chapter we called this *homeostasis*, or internal stability. In a tissue like the intestine, where the rate of cellular turnover is unusually high, control of programmed cell death becomes especially important. The organ has to know how many cells to make to replace the quickly dead and dying so that the life-giving intestine and colon function normally, processing food and waste, upon which the body relies. The onset of colorectal cancer occurs when this careful balance of cell death and replacement is disturbed.

We're going to proceed slowly now to help you fully understand the events that transpire molecularly and trigger the disease. As you might imagine, cellular changes take place in normal tissue that mutates into cancerous tissue in these vital organs. First, the normal cell layer on the surface of the intestine and colon progresses to a highly specialized "overgrown" state. Think back on the car pile-ups at the large pothole site described earlier in this chapter. As cars pile up, resulting in hyperplasia, this overgrowth takes the form of polyps or mounds of cells protruding into the intestine. Some of these polyps can then advance to early adenomas (pronounced *"ADD-ee-NOME-ahs"*), or a benign tumor in a secretory gland like the intestine. The benign tumor exists in a pre-cancerous state, but it can advance to intermediate and late-stage adenomas on the twisted path toward cancer. When a late-stage adenoma progresses to a carcinoma, full colorectal cancer is present. But what molecular events trigger the steps up this ladder from polyps to adenomas to colorectal carcinomas?

As mentioned, there are dozens of cancer-initiating genes associated with the various organs and tissues of the body. With respect to colorectal cancer, a mutation in the gene known as APC triggers the disease, causing cells of the normal intestinal wall to form pre-cancerous polyps. APC produces a vital protein, and when it mutates, that protein is rendered flawed and non-functional. While APC is not one of the usual gatekeepers associated with the onset of uncontrolled cell growth, it bears all the characteristics of a gatekeeper when the mutation occurs in the colorectal region of the body. As far as cells of the intestinal wall are concerned, APC is indeed a gatekeeper. It doesn't tote a spray can of lubricant like mechanic proteins described in the second chapter. A mutant APC gums up everything and causes the cells of the intestinal wall to become more "sticky." The stickier the cells get, the longer they remain on the surface of the intestine instead of being "shed." That causes a dangerous imbalance in the delicate cell cycle of this vital bodily region, because these rapidly dividing and accumulating cells eventually become polyps and later, adenomas. If these "bad" cells were sloughed off, as they should, if the APC gene were not malfunctioning, no growth would occur.

But there's more bad news about imbalance when a mutation occurs in the APC gene. A healthy gene of this type makes a product that normally suppresses the manufacture of yet another genetic commodity, a protein called COX-2. This protein is as essential as the driver, the gatekeeper capsule D explained in the second chapter. When the driver is produced in overabundance, pre-cancerous conditions can occur. Essentially that's what happens when APC genes malfunction, allowing COX-2 proteins to skyrocket to unusually high levels, causing yet another imbalance in the colorectal system.

Here's how it occurs. Recent evidence suggests that COX-2 stimulates cell proliferation and also blocks the normal mechanisms of programmed death in cells of the intestinal wall. In other words, cells do not die as orderly as they should when a mutation affects this protein. As we have mentioned, in the colorectal region, programmed cell death and growth literally hold your life in the balance. Both have to be maintained precisely at proper levels. So it is not surprising that the cell-death inhibitor, COX-2, can greatly influence cellular expansion within the intestine. Neither is it surprising that hyperplasia develops when a malfunctioning APC gene gums up the intestinal wall and doesn't produce a substance to control COX-2, leading to an overabundance of that protein—and, as a result, longer lifespans for certain cells associated with the colorectal region. As new cells are made, in response to the mutation, pre-cancerous polyps develop. Moreover, this analysis also illustrates why cancer is a class of diseases rather than one disease. While COX-2 and APC cause pre-cancerous conditions in the colorectal region, they may not be involved in other cancers at all. The formation of tumors within any tissue depends ultimately upon the special biology of that tissue. But all such tumors have one thing in common: genetic mutations and subsequent damage to the cell cycle. That's why envisioning the process being described throughout this chapter will empower your consciousness so that you will be able to understand the basic functions that lead to any type of cancer.

At this point, with respect to colorectal cancer, we have described only part of the process—how APC mutation leads to pre-cancerous polyps and benign tumors. There's a stretch yet to go along the twisted path to full-blown cancer. While polyps and early adenomas usually only show mutations in APC, intermediate—or more advanced adenomas—begin to show mutations in another gene called RAS. Let's compare APC with RAS so that you can understand why this second mutation in the RAS gene is associated with more advanced cases.

As we mentioned, the APC gene makes a product that suppresses the COX-2 protein. However, the product of a malfunctioning APC gene does not have that effect on COX-2 and can lead to pre-cancerous tissue in the colorectal region. As such, though, APC is not directly connected to the cell cycle. The gene RAS *is* directly connected. RAS also strongly influences the four gatekeepers described in previous chapters and is one of the most common of the 100 or more associated "oncogenes," or cancer-causing genes.

To envision RAS, think of a carrier pigeon on a fencepost. It actually perches on the outer membrane of cells and can be triggered into action—dispatched to deliver its message—when it spots molecules that signal cell growth. The message is then delivered, and we discussed in earlier chapters what happens then, concerning the gatekeeper known as cyclin D, or the "driver," which plays a key role in signaling new cell growth. Cells with large amounts of RAS on their surface are unusually sensitive to these growth signals. They release messages which, ultimately, produce more "drivers" that stimulate cells to divide faster. An intestinal cell with both an APC and a RAS mutation has both an enhanced cell cycle and a blocked cell death program, a dubious combination. Daughter cells replicate ever more quickly, and offspring that should have short lifespans now are "sticky" and have longer ones. The result is mass of tissue: a tumor.

Now we come to late-stage adenomas, developing ever closer to full blown cancer of the colon. As you might anticipate by now, knowing the vagaries of mutations, late-stage adenomas are triggered by yet another mutation—this time in a gene called DCC. When operating properly, this gene acts like the gatekeeper suppressor, "p53," (described by its atomic weight). But when the DCC gene mutates, suppression of cell division breaks down, as if jammed by radar. By now, the accumulation of mutations, from APC to RAS to DCC, triggers wild cell replication. All this leads to a mutation in the enzyme that initiates DNA repair, or the monitoring and fixing of errors association with cell replication.

By now the twisted path of pre-cancer is beginning to approach cancer. At the molecular level all hell is breaking loose on the once smooth roadway where the first large pothole appeared. More and more cars are streaming down that surface, piling up in accidents. More and more potholes are being spotted along the route, resulting in greater pile-ups. And street repair is becoming near impossible because the cars—cells that keep replicating because of an overabundance of "drivers" and other oncogenes—seemingly are coming from nowhere. The once stable cellular neighborhood appears increasingly disorderly. Finally, as more and more cars hit potholes and pile up in an increasing mass of tissue constituting a still benign but late-stage tumor, the specter of cancer approaches ever so much nearer.

The neighborhood is in disrepair because of several genetic misfires: faulty DNA repair and subsequent over-activation of the cell cycle, because of mutants and ineffective suppression and cell-death programming. In a word, it's the beginning of the end for intestinal cells harboring these mutations. And the end soon arrives with a mutation in the gatekeeper suppressor, sparking the onset of colorectal carcinoma. **Figures 8 through 12** show the steps in the progression towards colorectal cancer and the mutations associated with these steps. But while the sequence of steps shown in these diagrams is often the sequence of mutations leading to colorectal cancer, this disease can result from these mutations happening in a very different sequence. This is merely an example of how a specific cancer progresses from an initial single mutational 'hit' to full cancer. Again, however, your understanding the process is the point of this case study.

❧ ❧ ❧

A Likely Chain of Events

Information presented here is basic. Mutations and their sequences vary, depending on the specific cancer and cellular biology and cycles from which the various cancers originate. However, several general mutational events occur in almost all cancers, allowing their continued progression. Any attempt to describe cancer needs to include a discussion of at least three of these general mutational changes associated with the disease.

A tumor requires certain conditions to survive. Again, situations vary and involve a host of proteins and oncogenes. But one general requirement involves mutations within a cancer cell, thus letting the defective cell circumvent its death program. Another condition is stealth. This occurs at the molecular level when specific alterations are made in any population of flourishing cancer cells, allowing them to avoid immune surveillance

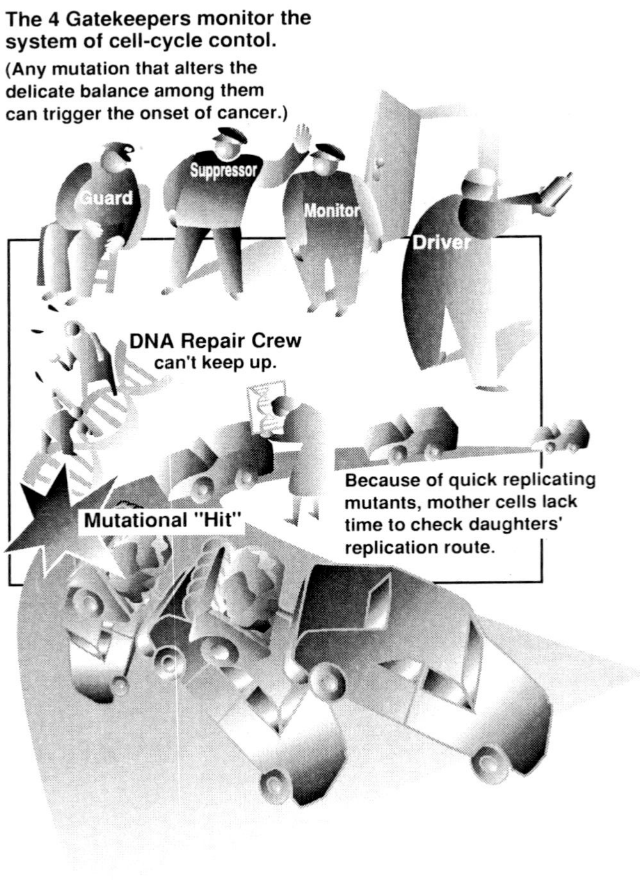

Figure 8.
Genetic mistakes are dramatic, condeming every other "cell"-mother traveling the stretch of DNA to spiral out of control at the original "accident" site, or mutation. Hyperplasia developes as car upon car piles up here.

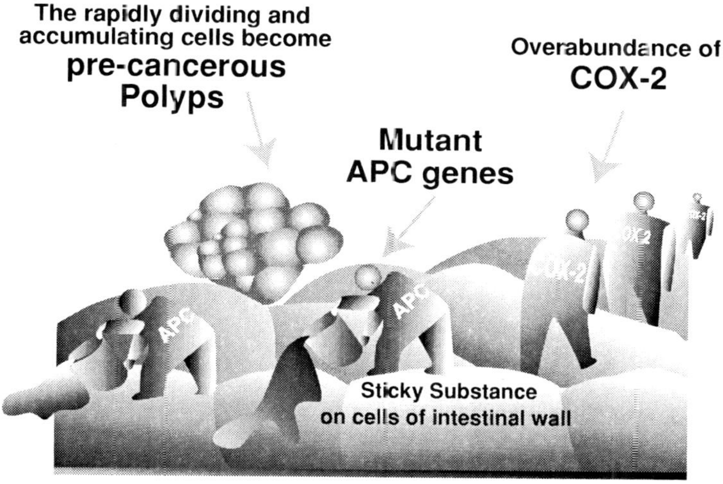

Figure 9.
Malfunctioning APC genes gum up the intestinal wall and do not produce a substance to control the cell-death inhibitor called COX-2. As new cells are made, in response to the mutation, pre-cancerous polyps develop.

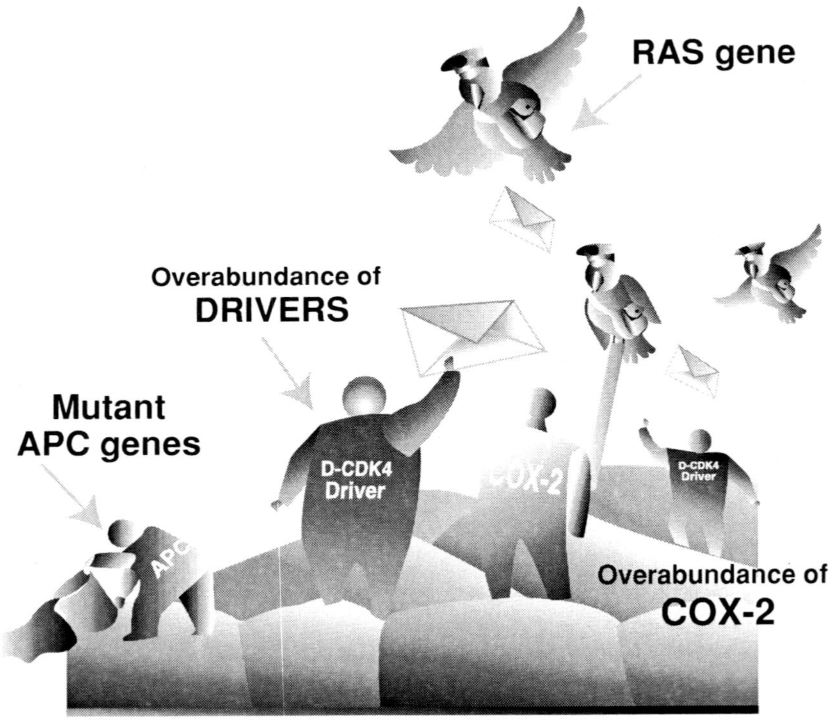

Figure 10.
RAS "carrier pigeons" release more and more messages that produce an overabundance of "drivers," stimulating cells to divide faster.

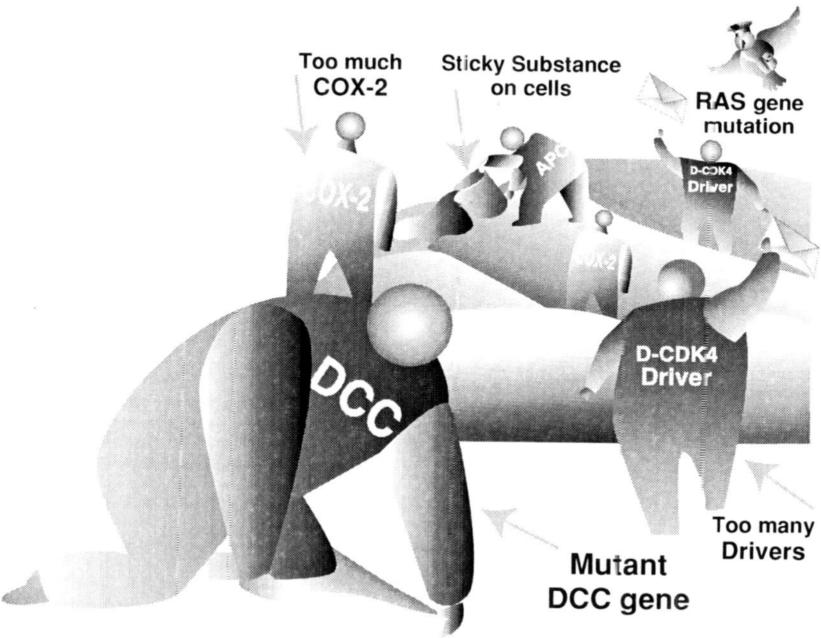

Figure 11.
When the DCC gene mutates, cell suppression ceases. The disruption allows cells to multiply wildly.

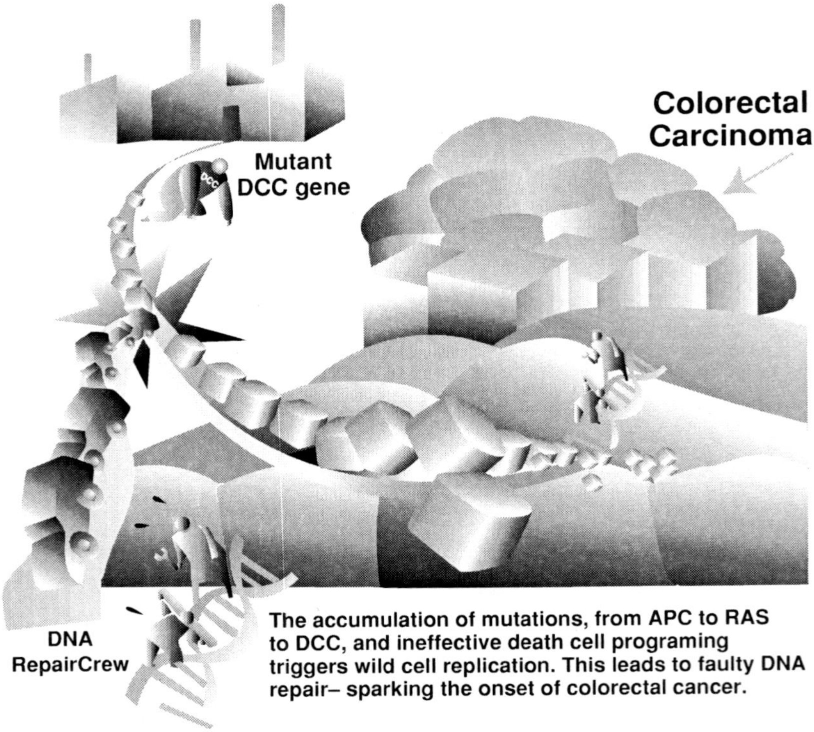

Figure 12.
The end soon arrives with a mutation in the gatekeeper suppressor, sparking the onset of colorectal carcinoma.

that might otherwise eradicate them naturally. Just like any other living organism, even the sublime monster of cancer requires food. The increasing mass of cells in an expanding tumor must have access to a plentiful supply of nutrients to maintain its growth. To accomplish this, the cells of the tumor must engineer the production of a system of blood vessels to "feed" the growing cancer. So as you can see, although the illustrations in **Figures 8 through 12** show the progression from one mutational hit to full-blown cancer, other processes are occurring in the body. The three molecular events described here—escape from programmed cell death, stealth from natural immune forces, and construction of blood vessels—are also vital steps along the path from pre-cancer to full blown cancer.

The phenomenon of programmed cell death is a partner of cell-cycle control. The death and replication programs must work in tandem to maintain a constant number of cells within each tissue. But programmed death also serves another important function in the cellular neighborhood. Throughout the complex workings of the cell many sensors carefully monitor all aspects of cellular function and inspect the cellular machinery that performs those functions. When monitor proteins recognize any significant breakdown or damage to the critical molecules of the cell, they signal the action proteins of the cell-death program to begin terminating the suspect cell. These powerful action proteins then chew up and destroy the cell's proteins and its DNA before causing the cell to fragment into blebs, harmless microscopic "bubbles." Moreover, because the most important of all the cell's molecules is its DNA, the double helix is continually monitored for excessive damage. While small errors in the DNA's message are corrected by the DNA repair system, larger damage should trigger rapid destruction of the cell to stop the propagation and perpetration of gross genetic errors.

We've discussed how serious damage to the cellular neighborhood ensues. The cell loses control of its cycle, begins to replicate wildly, and ceases to be able to monitor and repair its DNA efficiently. At this point, however, the DNA monitoring system should kick in and uncover significant damage, identifying the suspect cells and destroying them via the cell-death program. This mechanism is highly effective in the protection of the body against cancer. If the DNA monitoring system is working properly it will stop the progression of a precancerous condition before any real damage to the person has occurred.

The protein responsible for monitoring DNA damage plays a critical role in cellular surveillance. Guess which protein is assigned the job of monitoring the cell's DNA for excessive damage? It is one of our old gatekeeper friends, the suppressor protein "p53," which acts as one of the four controls of the cell cycle and which also activates the cell-death program when extensive DNA damage is observed (**see Figure 13**). If the gatekeeping suppressor has already been destroyed by the initial mutational "hit"—or by a subsequent mutation—one of the last safeguards offered by the cell-death program is lost forever, ensuring continued expansion of a hyperplasia, an adenoma, and/or a cancerous tumor.

You can now understand two factors involving the suppressor protein: One, it is found mutated and non-functional in a very high percentage of cancers. Two, mutational hits affecting the suppressor protein often represent the final step to full colorectal cancer. As such this gatekeeper protein can serve as an example of why cancer cells may be seen as "foreign" to the body's immune system and why the immune system offers yet another defense against cancer.

❧ ❧ ❧

The Role of the Immune System

Normally the immune system of the body recognizes invading agents like bacteria and viruses. The system can do this because foreign agents are made up of proteins different from the body's own "self-made" proteins. The way that our immune system can tell the difference between a "self" protein and a "foreign" protein is complex and difficult for biologists, let alone lay people to understand. Suffice it to say that such differentiation is an important aspect of immune function but is one that does not always work perfectly. Classic examples of the immune system going awry are provided by autoimmune diseases such as arthritis and lupus, where the body's immune system turns upon itself.

Cancer, as we've discussed, involves a defect in the cell cycle. Mutants are spawned, undermining the functions of gatekeepers like the suppressor. But the targets of these mutants are "self" proteins. Your body has created

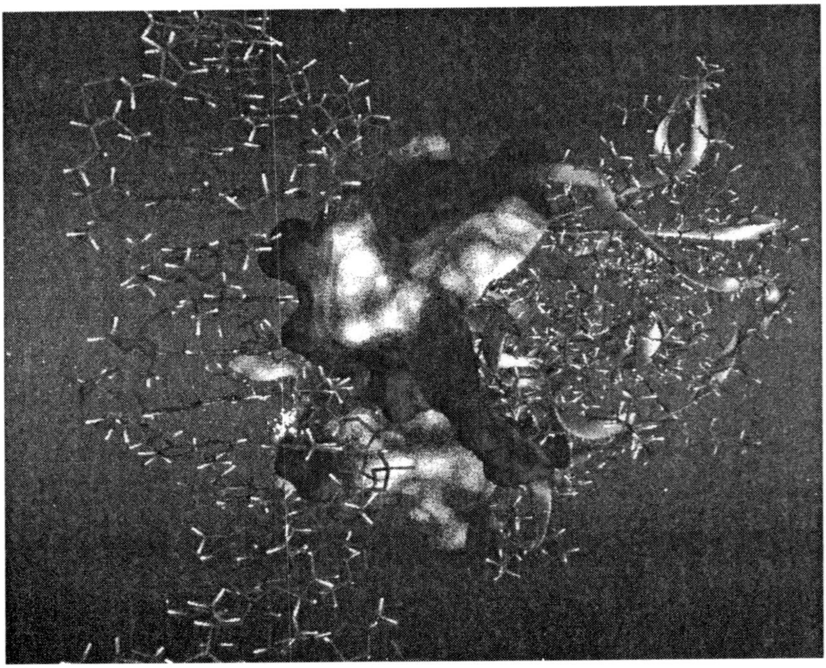

Figure 13.
A Gatekeeper at Work

The p53 suppressor protein binds to the promoter region of a gene, turning on its expression and suppressing cell replication.

(Special thanks to Professors Juergen A. W. Brickman and Matthias Keil of the Institut fuer Physikalische Chemie, Darmstadt University of Technology, Germany, for permission to use this photo.)

them, and so they are not always as readily detectable as bacteria, say. All this has influenced cancer research. Decades ago medical scientists discovered that some of the proteins of tumor cells stimulated an immune response. That was big news in the lab. Researchers were excited because they began to realize that the immune system could possibly be stimulated to attack a tumor and destroy it, just like it might destroy an invading virus or bacteria. The concept of tumor vaccines and vaccinations against cancer began to be discussed. But soon these same researchers became puzzled. They could not understand why the body's immune system often reacted against its own cells and proteins. Furthermore, they wondered why a cancer patient's tumor was not attacked by his or her own immune system.

The search for answers to these puzzling questions led to the discipline of tumor immunology. At first, researchers in this field thought that a mutational change in proteins like the gatekeepers made them appear foreign. To an extent, this was true. But the full answer to this question proves to be much more complex and remains unanswered. Since the suppressor protein is mutated in such a high percentage of human cancers, it has become a primary concern of tumor immunologists. But they have demonstrated that its foreign appearance to the

❖ Inspiration Point

It is likely that many pre-cancerous growths within our bodies are cleared away by our immune systems. Thus, cancer has to overcome this obstacle to establish itself within the body. With each passing day, we are learning more ways to bolster the immune system in the fight against cancer.

body's immune system is not necessarily due to its mutated chemistry. When the suppressor is mutated and can no longer stop or slow cell replication, the out-of-control cell—trying to "heal" or correct errors—calls for more and more of this particular gatekeeper. It's as if residents of the cellular neighborhood in crisis put in a massive 911-emergency call, requesting suppressors. But instead of healthy, law-abiding officers of the molecular community, mutant gatekeepers show up. So even though dramatically increased levels of the suppressor are produced in the pre-cancer cell, they can do nothing to stop replication because the mutated gatekeeper no longer can suppress cell division. Yet cells keep crying for more. For this reason, vastly higher levels of the "p53" suppressor protein are present in cancer and pre-cancerous cells than in normal cells.

The suppressor is a key player in maintaining cellular health. In normal cells, the suppressor is produced in extremely small amounts that go instantly to the cell's nucleus and bind to the genes, one of which directs the manufacture of another gatekeeper, the "p21" monitor. Each of the few suppressor molecules present in a normal cell are tightly bound to DNA and closeted away within the realm of the cell's genes. Contemporary immunologists are beginning to wonder if the immune system ever really "sees" any suppressor proteins in a normal cell. Perhaps genetic signaling proteins like the suppressor are never effectively observed by the body's immune system and are never categorized as "self." Perhaps this explains why high levels of the suppressor suddenly appearing within cancer cells seem "foreign" to the immune system. But if that is so, why doesn't the immune system attack these cells and clear them from the body? After all, the body is now full of this apparently foreign protein.

It is quite likely that many pre-cancerous growths within our bodies are, indeed, cleared away by our immune systems. As such, cancer has to overcome this obstacle to truly establish itself solidly within the body of an individual. But the challenge presented by the immune system can be surmounted by cancer cells, as long as they can rely on an accelerated cell cycle and impaired DNA repair. Among the frequent mutations occurring within such cells may be one that blocks the process by which the immune system recognizes and destroys a cell containing "foreign" proteins. Because such an individual cell is now rendered invisible to the immune challenge, it will seed a rapidly expanding population of like cells. These replicants know how to resist or circumvent the human immune system that normally protects our bodies from disease. As such, they represent yet another step along the twisted path toward malignant cancer. This route is probably a common one taken by almost all cancers.

It's important to understand how cancer cells might avoid the immune challenge. Our immune system does not "see" a foreign protein as a whole object, but only as small fragments of larger molecules. One way to describe the chemistry and structure of a protein molecule is to view it as a folded string of beads. A protein is a polymer of amino acids strung one after another like the beads on a necklace. The necklace of amino acids that makes up a protein is not stretched out into a linear strand, but is folded back and forth upon itself to generate a complex three dimensional structure. Thousands of these complex structures make up the architecture of life itself, and the design is as awe-inspiring as any creation by master architects Frank Lloyd Wright or Buckminster Fuller.

The "eye" of our immune system does not behold these beautiful protein structures as unified entities in the same way that we behold magnificent buildings, however. In fact, our immune system does not even "see" proteins until after their demolition. The body's proteins are continually recycled by the remarkably efficient process of life. Worn proteins are broken down by the recycling factories of the cell, first into fragments and then further into their component amino acids. The recyclers are known as "proteosomes" (pronounced *"PRO-tee-oh-sohms"*), which process fragments into short segments of a necklace. These fragments usually contain only 10 or fewer beads of an otherwise long protein chain. Our immune system recognizes proteins by these recycled fragments. Every cell of the body contains a very special protein that "presents" them.

Let's use an Asian metaphor to illustrate these special proteins. They hold their tiny fragments much the same way that an ancient Japanese woman might present a gift to a Samurai warlord. The women might appear "delicate" holding their beaded gifts, but they are powerfully in league with the warlords and inform them when to attack. The women grasp the beaded strands in clefts of microscopic, outstretched "hands." They do this on the surface of every cell, adorning them with the tell-tale fragments of recycled proteins. The warlords approach and inspect each cell to see if shards of any foreign proteins are among its decorations. If the warring white blood cells find any such foreign fragments, they attack and destroy that cell. Before the warriors strike, however, they must also engage other associated proteins that activate the attack plan. If a cell dividing wildly and amassing mutants experiences a "hit" in the gene encoding either the "presenting" protein or any of her partners—destroying any of their abilities to perform—that cell has mastered "stealth." It becomes invisible to the immune defenses of the body. The warlord approaches, inspects the woman's beaded chain, and cannot discern anything amiss. In this way most cancers avoid being cleared from the body by the immune system. Like the mutations blocking the programmed death of aberrant cells, mutations rendering a cell invisible to the immune system allow that cell to propagate and expand into unchecked cancer.

The Final Step to Cancer

Once an initial mutation obliterates cell-cycle control and additional mutations, like those discussed above, elude the immune system, there is but one final step before these cancer cells can overtake the body: the tumor's continuing need for a food source to feed its growing mass. If sufficient nutrients cannot be found the growing tumor will simply die of starvation. So, as we see in all of biology—from the mammoth whale to the infinitesimal mutant—*food matters*.

❖ Inspiration Point

A tumor, like any other body part, has a continuing need for a food source to feed its growing mass. If sufficient nutrients cannot be found, the tumor will simply die of starvation. This concept is at the root of such new therapies involving *angiogenesis inhibition*.

Cells receive nutrients via a complex system of blood vessels and tiny branching capillaries. In order for such a system to form around and throughout an expanding tumor, the cells of that tumor must produce protein "factors"—biological entities associated with a chemical or biophysical process—in this case, the stimulation of the growth of blood vessels. These factors are not normally produced by tumor cells. As you may recall, this means that the regulatory regions of these genes do not naturally activate the production of such factors in tumor cells. So the tumor just keeps growing until the existing neighboring blood vessels can no longer supply enough nutrients. The most essential nutrient supplied solely by the tumor's diminishing blood supply is oxygen, life's sustaining gas. Tumors need oxygen to survive, just as we do. Deprived of oxygen, tumor cells "starve" and die—again, just as we do. When tumor cells lack a sufficient oxygen supply, they trigger the activation of genes and through a molecular process stimulate the sprouting and growth of new blood vessels to supply life-giving oxygen and other nutrients to the starving tumor. This response is natural to life. It is an aspect of all our body's cells, not only tumor cells. If your finger is severely cut, severing the blood supply to your fingertip, that fingertip lacks oxygen and signals an emergency. The oxygen deficiency within the cells of your fingertip activates those genes that now produce factors that stimulate the repair and regrowth of these severed blood vessels after you bandage your cut finger. Tumors require more oxygen because they expand and have more mass and so simply use this natural repair mechanism to solve their problem of diminishing nutrient and oxygen supply. When a tumor gets enough oxygen and other nutrients, it continues to expand because it can stimulate the formation of a system of blood vessels to feed *itself*.

That's bad enough. Such a tumor can expand indefinitely. But the cancer still cannot spread from the tumor to other tissues and metastasize until yet another mutation or series of mutations occurs. That's because cells of *like tissues*—two intestinal cells, for example—have similar surface molecules that allow them to stick to each other and forbid them from sticking to the cells of other tissues. This feature of cellular biology is an oft-overlooked wonder of nature, for without it, we would smolder into protoplasmic blobs. *So tumors of one tissue cannot spread to another tissue unless they mutate these surface proteins.* And by now this is a distinct possibility because the cancer has its own sublime bio-intelligence. Given time, it might figure all this out. Once it does, the tumor may spread throughout the body. After these final mutations have taken place, the enemy within is now a rapidly growing malignant tumor that has already begun to spread throughout the body, threatening the patient's life.

❧ ❧ ❧

A Moment of Reflection

Let's step back a moment and consider just how long cancer has taken to proceed from its first mutational hit to its ultimate end. By understanding the process, already you will have busted one of cancer's most powerful myths—one that can target your consciousness as a mutant targets a gatekeeper—and that is, that cancer occurs spontaneously as if a demon has waved a mystical wand. Make no mistake about these myths. While busting them cannot heal cancer, they certainly can ease pain. You will recall how, at the beginning of this chapter, Michael Bugeja's mother—afflicted by Mediterranean myth—believed cancer was as contagious as leprosy and forbade her father from a loving last encounter with his grandchild. Ask yourself, how might "Pop" have faired in the cancer ward of the 1950s if he not only had that last loving encounter but also the support and tenderness of personal "factors," a network of compassionate and informed friends, relatives, and hospital personnel. Ask yourself as well, knowing the twisted path that pre-cancer must take before becoming cancer, how important medical checkups truly are in the early detection of this disease. True,

> **❖ Inspiration Point**
>
> **Knowing the path that pre-cancer must take before becoming cancer, you should realize the importance of medical checkups. Such detection may lead to the words—"you have cancer"; but with new treatments available, you might also hear: "There's good news."**

early detection may lead to the words—"you have cancer"; but with new treatments available or forthcoming, you might also learn: "There's good news." Consider how knowledge has empowered you already, after less than half of this book. By now you can see that cancer is as much a disease of accumulated mutations as it is a disease of the cell cycle. Moreover, you now know dozens of medical and biogenetic terms associated with cancer. Perhaps you are lucky enough to be checked or treated by a physician who thoroughly explains every technical detail, symptom, and diagnosis. Chances are, however, that your doctor lacks the time. And doctors are used to patients knowing little about cancer treatment and prevention, especially at the molecular level. How might he or she respond when you can discuss this disease with the scientific perspective being shared here? True, the result may be that the physician might feel intimidated and abruptly end the discussion. If so, you might benefit by seeking out more compassionate care. A more probable scenario, however, is that the attending physician will not only respect your knowledge, sharing more information instead of bedside clichés, but may also be inspired by your acumen, taking special interest in your case and/or learning more about it.

Knowledge really is power. It busts myth and undermines fear associated with cancer. It also gives you a sense of control, the very thing that a mutant destroys with respect to cellular functions and that cancer destroys with respect to bodily functions. That's part of the sublime, the confined space that opens to expanse, as explained in the epigraph at the beginning of this chapter by the great mythologist Joseph Campbell. As he knew, knowledge of the sublime allows us to view a monster like a mutant with a steady, compassionate gaze, expanding consciousness and further eroding fear.

The sublime is at the heart of all great art and at the root of scientific inspiration. Einstein called the latter "rapturous amazement at the harmony of natural law." The sublime imparts elegant, transcendent truths, even about haunting images, so that we can acknowledge the beautiful in the ugly and vice versa. As any art historian will tell you, knowledge of the sublime enhances perception. After all, the concept of the sublime is one of the most ancient in Occidental culture. Scholars have had trouble pegging the original writer of *On the Sublime* and only recently have credited a first-century Greek intellect named Dionysius Longinus for the insightful book.

Longinus describes the sublime as "the sound of greatness," moral and imaginative, that emanates from deep within. A person able to perceive the sublime experiences thoughts of grandeur even about topics that typically evoke terror and horror in society. It's important to know, as Longinus believed, that the sublime is not confined to epic events or grand concepts. It is also found in ordinary events in any age.

The sublime deals with two types of archetypal truths: epiphanies and peak experiences. An epiphany is a moment of clarity in which your *mind* is at one with the universe. A peak experience occurs when your *body* is at one with the universe. Expansive truths emanate from such seemingly ordinary events: a divorce, a birth, a disease. You wake up early one morning and know the precise incident that eventually led to estrangement. Or you realize the sublime "pain" of childbirth, your (or a spouse's) body creating out of DNA a new life form and subsequent consciousness. The following envisioning exercise is designed to help you "experience the sublime" and thus help reduce your fear of cancer.

❦ ❦ ❦

Envisioning Exercise

Experience the Sublime

Objective: To confront your memory and feelings about cancer—inspiring you to experience "the sublime," reducing your fear about cancer.

For this exercise, contemplate the questions and write answers to them in your journal. Or, you may tape record your thoughts. As another alternative, you may ponder these questions until you clearly imagine them coming to life.

1. What is your earliest memory about cancer?

2. Who were the people involved?

3. Where did the scene take place?

4. To the best of your knowledge, what was each person feeling at the time?

5. What epiphany and/or peak experience is associated with this memory?

6. What fear is attached to the memory?

7. How might truth and knowledge put the fear into perspective?

While you may start with your earliest memory of cancer, you don't have to restrict yourself to this earliest memory. You can contemplate other events surrounding the high and low points of your life with respect to cancer. When you do so, you will have compiled many anecdotes about the role that cancer has played in your life. Feel free to convey these stories to others—you will see how even strangers share many of your experiences and personal truths. Like a Japanese temple opening out to a beautific horizon, you will experience the sublime. When you do, focus your steady gaze on the genetic monster known as cancer whose power and awe command your respect and attention . . . but should not fearfully consume your consciousness.

Chapter Five

❦ ❦ ❦

Lessons from the AIDS Virus

Concerning all acts of initiative there is one elementary truth, the ignorance of which kills countless ideas and splendid plans: that the moment one definitely commits oneself, then Providence moves too. All sorts of things occur to help one that would have otherwise never have occurred. A whole stream of events issues from the decision, raising in one's favor all manner of unforeseen incidents and meetings and material assistance, which no one could have dreamt would have come their way.

—W. H. Murray (1913-1996),
leader of the Scottish Himalayan Expedition, 1951

❧ ❧ ❧

The following is another recollection of co-author Michael Bugeja:

Since childhood, I dreamed of becoming a writer. At age 24, I got my chance. I had just finished a master's degree in mass communications in South Dakota when I learned about a six-month position to help cover the Legislature in Pierre for United Press International. Finally it looked like my dream was coming true—at least for a short while. It was 1975, and journalism had reached the height of its popularity. The country had just suffered through impeachment proceedings against President Richard Nixon, who resigned, yielding the office to President Gerald Ford. Like most aspiring reporters, I had a vision of being an award-winning investigative journalist—like Bob Woodward or Carl Bernstein, the Washington Post *reporters who cracked the Watergate break-in story. Now I was working for UPI, one of the most powerful media outlets in the world. The problem, though, was that I had six months to investigate and report a story as powerful as the Pulitzer Prize-winning series by Woodward and Bernstein.*

I had already been told that there was no chance—no chance, my editor told me on my first day—that I would get a permanent job with UPI. The wire service was losing money.

There were threats of strikes and massive lay-offs. Worse, as a new reporter I was not going to get exciting assignments. My job was to make coffee, answer phones, do the daily weather and cattle market reports, and rewrite an occasional public relations release.

The dream of a blockbuster story was rapidly becoming a nightmare. To work in a major newsroom, to be so close to the action—watching reporters rushing in and out with hot news stories, listening to the continual tin background music of the teletype—and not to be part of it, devastated the cub reporter with Pulitzer dreams.

After two weeks, I decided to forget the dreams of the past and goals of the future and just enjoy each day of my remaining time in the UPI newsroom. In college, I despised the drudgery of rewriting PR releases, those poorly written attempts to generate publicity or inspire public service. I felt my time was too valuable to waste doing that. But now I vowed to adopt a positive attitude, relishing the moment and setting a standard of excellence for myself, so that I could enjoy each precious day as a reporter. So if I was assigned to rewrite a news release, then I would excel at this otherwise mundane task. In sum, I had made a commitment to excellence.

On the top of the pile of news releases that day was one from the Department of Communicable Diseases in the Health Department, noting the percent of the population of South Dakota that had been inoculated with the swine flu vaccine. In 1975, the Ford administration had ordered a national inoculation program to ward off what some predicted would be a catastrophic epidemic in this country. Each state was trying to vaccinate all of its citizens, and the percentage rate was routine news. I read the PR release and noted that it was dated a week earlier, one of those boring tasks that I had put off as long as I could, hoping that my editor would assign me a real news story. Since I had made my commitment, I decided to act on it and visit the Health Department personally, to get a few quotes from an official, along with an updated percentage.

The first person I met was a secretary. I asked, "What's new with the swine flu vaccination program?" And she answered, "The damn thing is causing paralysis."

That encounter led to my top news story as a journalist. Armed with the secretary's tip, I was the first to report that the swine flu vaccine could trigger Guillain-Barre syndrome, a temporary paralysis that causes muscle weakness and inflammation of nerve roots. Reporters across the country quickly followed up on my initial accounts, ending the inoculation program and earning the cub reporter—you guessed it—a permanent job with United Press International. In three years, I became state editor for North and South Dakota, and credited my success to commitment and a change in attitude. And just as William Hutchinson Murray promised, a whole stream of events ensued from that initial decision, "raising in one's favor all manner of unforeseen incidents and meetings and material assistance, which no one could have dreamt would have come their way."

❧ ❧ ❧

Taming A Deadly Epidemic

There was another killer epidemic in the 1980s: AIDS. Hearing that prognosis back then was worse than hearing the word "cancer." To have AIDS (Acquired Immune Deficiency Syndrome) was to be sentenced to death. No one would have dreamed that in less than a decade, real progress would be made in the fight against AIDS. By 1996, researchers were able to better monitor and control the AIDS virus in patients infected by HIV (*human immunodeficiency virus*). Because of this first real breakthrough, many HIV-infected patients enjoyed dramatic improvements in overall health. Since 1996 more discoveries have occurred, but this early one made a lasting impression on geneticists. The breakthrough was achieved because of an observation about the virus and its stealthy ability to elude detection. Before the discovery, there was growing suspicion among AIDS researchers that far more HIV virus particles were sequestered within the lymph nodes of infected patients than previously thought.

Lymph is a pale fluid associated with the immune system. It bathes bodily tissues and carries off bacteria, viruses and other particles to the *nodes*—a complex network of microscopic "mesh." The mesh impedes the passage of these foreign objects. In response, cells called lymphocytes (pronounced *"LIMPH-oh-SITES"*) proliferate, some of which produce other cells and molecules that attack the foreign particles. While AIDS and cancer differ, especially with respect to treatment, they share one basic commonality: *mutations*.

AIDS, like cancer, has an ability to form *multiple mutations*. When it does, it masters stealth and can elude the immune system for a period of time. Researchers who first analyzed HIV-positive patients were baffled because they didn't detect much virus. So they thought that HIV was a "slow" virus, taking years to express itself as AIDS. As they analyzed their research more carefully, they saw that the virus had accumulated in the lymph nodes. Moreover, it wasn't a "slow" virus.

Here's how those researchers made this discovery. They did a rigorous mathematical analysis of the interplay between virus replication—how the HIV multiplied and spread—and its elimination by the body's defenses. The results were startling. Study after study argued convincingly that an astoundingly high level of viral replication occurred in all HIV-infected patients, allowing the virus to persist for a prolonged period of infection and eventually evade immune surveillance and drug therapy. At a critical point, the virus would result in AIDS . . . just as a late-stage adenoma results in cancer, though by a different cellular process. In any case, between one hundred million and one billion HIV viruses were found to be produced each day in infected patients. But researchers also determined that nearly this same number of viruses were being cleared each day by the

❖ Inspiration Point

Scientists and ethicists accept truth as they find it, even if it goes against everything they hitherto have believed. They know that facts always lead to broader truths and that, in turn, leads to new discoveries or solutions . . . as happened in the fight against AIDS.

body's immune system. That's why they were initially mistaken, believing that AIDS was a slow virus. In retrospect, the clearance of viruses from the body by the immune system shows how efficient that system actually is. But time wears it down, partly because of the sheer number of viruses it has to remove each day. Nonetheless, this prolonged balance between virus production and clearance explained the long period of apparent latency in HIV disease between infection and the onset of AIDS. But it also exposed the real seeds of disaster, revealing how HIV leads to AIDS over the prolonged period.

Again, the culprit is mutation. Even an HIV infected patient who shows no signs of disease can harbor a million distinct mutations of the HIV virus. Worse, an AIDS patient may harbor as many as a billion such variants as a result of mutations occurring at rapid frequency during HIV replication. In the absence of drug therapy, these mutants produce a cadre of viral variants that elude immune surveillance and expand at alarming rates. The virus is so aggressive that it can spawn mutations to resist a single drug therapy in a sheer matter of weeks or less.

That fact, while disheartening, led to effective treatment. And there's a lesson here for the layperson about the power of consciousness, courage, and reason. Scientists and ethicists share common ground when it comes to news as disturbing as the aggressiveness of the AIDS virus: *They accept the truth, no matter how unfair or unlikely, even if that truth goes against everything they have hitherto believed.* Science and ethics also share the same ultimate goal: seeing the world as it actually is, rather than through personal filters as we would want it to be. The reason is simple: Once you know key facts about anything from viruses to virtues, you can rely on consciousness to discover other facts that lead to a broader, more universal truth or to the resolution of a problem. But you have to gaze unflinchingly at the truth, and that takes courage. The greater the courage, the steadier the gaze—even at the molecular level. AIDS researchers knew this, envisioning the cellular terrain and relying on reason to outsmart HIV, a deadly and stealthy virus.

Here's how they did it. They analyzed the disturbing news about the high mutation rate associated with HIV replication. They knew that the virus was as lethal as the "Borg," those science-fiction *Star Trek* mutant life-forms able to mutate and overcome any one weapon, however powerful, used against them in galactic battles. Microscopic battles are fought regularly in the body, also. AIDS researchers observed the tactics of HIV, a formidable "alien" viral army assembling against healthy cells on the molecular landscape. So they switched strategies, suggesting not one elixir-like drug but multiple drug therapies to erect a barrier to HIV replication so high, barbed, and complex that the virus would not be able to mutate around it. These researchers reasoned that while a single virus could easily mutate around any one drug, the virus would find it exceedingly difficult or impossible to mutate around several different drugs at the same time.

❧ ❧ ❧

A Three-Pronged Attack

Effective AIDS treatment boiled down to basic mathematics and the power of reason to outsmart aggressive organisms. To elude a cocktail of drug-induced barriers, researchers theorized, HIV would have to experience several mutations in different genes *at the same time.* If these multiple mutations did not occur together, any virus that had mutated around one drug would still be instantly destroyed by the other drugs. Scientists did not know of any virus able to spawn simultaneous *multiple* mutations, so they felt that manifold drug therapy might actually halt the HIV infection. Because of the logic of their argument, physicians began treating patients with HIV disease and AIDS with a combination of two known drugs and also a new class of potent HIV protease (pronounced *"PRO-tee-ase"*) inhibitors.

Protease is any enzyme that can chop other proteins into fragments. Imagine a platoon of plastic miniature "Army men," those popular toy soldiers connected at the base by another strip of plastic. Typically parents use scissors to snip off each soldier so a child can play with them. Likewise, protease acts as scissors, separating each soldier from a "plastic" strip of microscopic tissue—in effect, rendering that "soldier" (in this case, HIV virus)—active to fight. When protease is inhibited, however, the viral platoon cannot operate at all.

In effect, researchers had lobbed a triple weapon at HIV. The combination of two drugs attacking one part of the viral machinery and protease inhibitors attacking the other brought about significant progress in infected patients. Many patients who can tolerate such treatments have since enjoyed significant improvement in overall health. One in particular has been basketball great Earvin "Magic" Johnson, one of the early patients to receive the triple drug therapy, which his personal physician, Dr. David Ho of the Aaron Diamond AIDS Research Center in New York, helped to develop.

> **❖ Inspiration Point**
>
> **Effective AIDS treatment boiled down to basic mathematics and the power of reason to outsmart a virus as aggressive as a cancerous tumor. In part because of AIDS research, new approaches and therapies are evolving to treat cancer.**

Dr. Ho may be partly responsible for transforming public perception about AIDS, no longer an automatic death sentence. In fact, some physicians believe that Ho's triple therapy may render AIDS as manageable as diabetes. Nonetheless, Magic Johnson was lucky—not only in being Dr. Ho's patient—but also having his HIV infection detected during a routine blood test. The former NBA star believes his faith in God and prayers for good health account for low viral activity in his body. "If it wasn't for the Lord's blessing," he told a television reporter, "I wouldn't be as healthy as I am now." Although doctors and researchers credit Dr. Ho's therapy for the good results, they also note that Johnson is HIV-"*positive*" . . . in the attitudinal sense of that word. A positive attitude is medically associated with the placebo effect and, by extension, consciousness. However, soon after Johnson made his remarks about God's being responsible for his renewed health, a mini debate arose concerning science and religion: *Who, really, was responsible?*

In Magic Johnson's case, from a scientific standpoint, the factual answer is Dr. Ho, whose consciousness may have been God-inspired but whose research was grounded in natural laws. Scientists may feel, as Einstein did, that those laws evoke rapturous amazement, but God did not develop triple drug therapy. However, from a religious standpoint, it can be argued that prayers—at the very least—may have brought Dr. Ho and Magic Johnson together. And yet only the scientific explanation can be replicated in lab upon lab. Indeed, many patients pray desperately for cures or reliable treatment and, when their conditions worsen, deduce that they have been overlooked and/or abandoned by God. And that attitude hampers effective medical treatment. Thus, the ethical response to this science-vs.-religion debate is to avoid the debate altogether and accept the obvious harmony of groundbreaking research, potent medicine, and positive attitude in a willing patient. That's the triple "therapy" of this book.

❧ ❧ ❧

Focusing on the Process

Back to the triple drug therapy employed by Dr. Ho, who also noted that the virus strain found in an advanced AIDS patient may be markedly different from the virus strain that initiated the disease. That suggested vigorous multiple mutations. Thus, researchers began to realize—even in the first *partially* effective therapy for HIV disease—that focusing on the ultimate (or latest) viral strain may not be the best approach to achieve long-term results. So gradually they began to focus on the *process* of rapid mutation, analyzing how the virus survived in the body and overcame its natural defense mechanisms. We believe the insight gained from the study and treatment of HIV disease can help develop strategies for more effective treatments for other diseases, including cancer.

As discussed in earlier chapters, cancer is the result of:

- ❖ A defect in cell-cycle control.
- ❖ The selection of "survivor" cells from the myriad mutations resulting from this defect.
- ❖ Ineffective DNA repair, again hastened by mutations.

> **❖ Inspiration Point**
>
> **Physicians should know details of particular pre-cancerous or early stage cancer cells in order to choose an appropriate "cocktail" of therapeutic agents, erecting a multiple barrier to cancer's progression, much like Dr. David Ho did with AIDS when treating Earvin "Magic" Johnson.**

In many ways cancer is like AIDS in that it often lies in the body unnoticed for many years during which it accumulates the appropriate mutations necessary to allow its unchecked expansion and take-over of resources. At the moment cancer patients are treated by surgery, radiation and/or chemotherapy in an attempt to destroy the final selected form of the disease. Certainly this intervention has to continue since many cancers are not presented for treatment until they have reached this final stage. Moreover, new means to terminate final-stage cancer cells more effectively are being developed each year. But lessons learned from treatment of the AIDS virus suggest a very different approach to cancer therapy.

Perhaps the best opportunity to treat cancer—or any other illness associated with accumulated mutations—is early on in the progression of the disease, well before its final form has yet appeared. AIDS research also suggests the deployment of "multiple blockades" like triple-drug therapy, to outwit the mutation mathematically, slamming it with three or more lines of defense. If it morphs past one barrier, or even two, the next barrier will ensure its destruction. With respect to cancer, such an approach is based on three steps:

- Early detection by routine screening of pre-cancerous events, like polyps or adenomas.
- Detailed analysis of the molecular nature of any detected event.
- Use of simultaneous multiple approaches to treat it.

There is good news about early detection. Pre-cancerous events in the body are always associated with genetic mutations and with rapidly dividing cells. Extremely sensitive new DNA analysis methods, available through state-of-the-art "PCR" technology, allow the detection of mutations in the DNA of pre-cancerous cells . . . even if only a few are present in the body tissue being analyzed. That's vitally important, when you consider that this aid in treatment was unavailable only a few years ago. The undetected mutation could rely on an overpopulation of healthy cells to cloak its presence, part of the stealth that allowed it to replicate until eventually being spotted during a routine check-up, say. Research has also improved on the cellular level. For starters, mutations in certain genes (such as the gatekeeper suppresser) are found in a high percentage of precursors to most cancers, as explained in the last chapter. And soon most other genetic mutations associated with the onset of cancer will be known. Thus, the *targets* for sensitive PCR analysis are now also clear. After all, these mutations are associated with rapidly dividing cells that are often sloughed off tissues; so sampling body fluids can easily uncover them. The end result will be that doctors and researchers will know what to look for earlier on in the cancer process, thanks to knowledge empowered by new technology. And yet, simple detection may not be enough.

❖ Inspiration Point

Already a few advanced cancer treatment centers offer their patients a staff of physicians highly trained in the latest oncology procedures. These physicians are backed up by scientists trained in molecular biology, genetics, immunology and other aspects of cancer biology.

To apply the right barriers to slow or halt the expansion of precancerous tissue, physicians will need to know a few more facts. Which types of pre-cancers or early cancers are present? What mutations in which genes have already occurred? Think back to the last chapter, detailing steps from inception to the final stages of colorectal cancer. Such a progression of events occurs for each of the myriad cancers. First you have to identify the pre-cancerous tissue or an early stage of cancer in a patient. Then, to design or select therapeutic agents to block its progression, you have to know the *specific* mutations. Many of these new and exciting therapeutic approaches will be described in upcoming chapters. Some of these approaches are general for all forms of cancer. Others are highly specialized for cancers with certain existing genetic mutations. Nonetheless, the treating physician has to know details of the particular pre-cancerous or early stage cancer cells, to choose an appropriate "cocktail" of therapeutic agents, erecting a multiple barrier to cancer's progression, much like Dr. David Ho did with AIDS when treating Earvin "Magic" Johnson.

Likewise as in AIDS treatment, the triple approach of detection, analysis and multiple therapy is ideal not only for early stage disease but also for the final stage as well. This changes the treatment scenario for cancer patients of the near future. Instead of visiting a family physician and being referred to a specialist in oncology who thereafter would treat the patient alone, future patients most likely will be served by a complex group of physicians and medical scientists. Already a few advanced cancer treatment centers offer their patients a staff of physicians highly trained in the latest oncology procedures. These physicians are backed up by scientists trained in molecular biology, genetics, immunology and other aspects of cancer biology. Such teams of physicians and molecular scientists will soon become the norm for cancer treatment in the United States.

❧ ❧ ❧

The Future of Cancer Treatment

How, exactly, will such a therapy team function in the treatment of a cancer patient? We envision a new type of medical contingent, several years into the future, treating a patient. It wouldn't matter how a family physician detected the cancer. The doctor or patient could have located it as a solid tumor. Or the cancer may have been spotted during or after an X-ray, CAT scan, or Magnetic Resonance Imagery. In any case, the family physician would pinpoint the exact size of the tumor at a specific location. Then the patient would be referred to a surgical oncologist. The surgeon would quickly schedule a procedure during which he or she would biopsy the tumor, removing enough of the abnormal tissue so that both the pathologists and the allied cancer biologists could fully characterize and analyze the tumor. In some cases the preliminary pathology report might be completed while the patient remained in surgery. This way, the surgeon in the operating room could remove as much of the remaining cancerous tissue as possible. But in most cases the surgeon would close the patient as soon as the biopsy was finished and wait for a complete evaluation of the tumor before reaching a decision about doing more surgery.

Treatment, meanwhile, would continue. Now the cancer biologists would swing into action. While pathologists were preparing slides to view the tumor cells under their microscopes, the molecular biologists would be preparing DNA from the cells of the biopsied tumor. With the patient recovering from surgery, small portions of the DNA from his or her tumor would already be transferred into many tiny plastic tubes used in sensitive PCR reactions to detect the tumor's accumulating mutations. These would be specifically identified before the next morning. Soon after, the pathologist, the molecular biologist and the surgeon would meet with the entire cancer therapy team and present their findings.

Like generals meeting in a war room, the physicians and scientists would map a strategy at this critical meeting. They would choose a therapy based on the type of tumor, the cell type of its origin, and the DNA mutations. This therapy might include surgery, excising the tumor; immunotherapy, enhancing the resistance of the immune system; radiation therapy, eradicating the tumor; gene therapy, transplanting genes into the cells to correct a defect; or advanced forms of chemotherapy, destroying the tumor. Except for the surgery, each of these therapeutic approaches would be specifically designed and targeted to the specific biology of the tumor generated by its unique array of accumulated mutations. Such future treatment not only would be highly specialized and focused on the tumor in question, but also would involve multiple agents to block any further mutations that may evade the therapy—again, a lesson learned from the AIDS virus.

There's one more puzzle piece missing from this future scenario about cancer treatment. It is a critical element needed to combat the disease: *a positive attitude,* requiring patients to make a commitment toward improved health, no matter what the prognosis or stage of illness. As mentioned earlier, mountaineer and author William Hutchinson Murray understood that as soon as a person commits to any endeavor, Providence will move, too.

> **❖ Inspiration Point**
>
> **In your private moments, make a new commitment to health awareness. Providence will move when you do.**

Murray never achieved the goal of scaling the Himalayans, by the way. He tried twice in 1950 and 1951 but could not acclimate to the altitude. He is remembered more as a writer than as a mountain climber, based on an act of Providence dating back to World War II, when he was captured by a tank commander in Africa after a fierce battle in which much of his platoon was wiped out. The commander took Murray at gunpoint, noticing that the prisoner was scantily clothed for the chilly desert night. The German officer asked him if he was cold, and Murray replied, "Cold as a mountain top!" Turns out that the officer was a mountain climber, too, and spared Murray's life, sending him to a prisoner of war camp. At that camp the Red Cross sent Murray a complete volume of Shakespeare and a roll of toilet paper. As the London *Guardian* newspaper put it, "The writer reversed the usual functions."

Murray wrote about mountain climbing in Scotland on that tissue roll. His first efforts were discovered and confiscated, but soon he was allowed to continue, and after the war his scribblings were typed up in manuscript form and published by Dent in 1947 under the title *Mountaineering in Scotland*. It is a literary/adventure classic to this day. To write it, Murray made a commitment to keep a positive attitude in the most dire of situations, a Nazi prisoner of war camp. To survive, he had to raise his consciousness to new levels of awareness. Below is an excerpt from another climbing book by Murray, *Undiscovered Scotland*:

> *"The full action of meditation is usually made difficult or impossible on mountains by wind and weather, time and company. But our observations can be made for later and more effective use in privacy. We should then recall the forms of beauty, visualizing each until our love for its beauty is aroused. . . . [I]t may be a sun rising or a sun setting, or a night sky or mountain, the beauty for which no words can be found. Encourage unreservedly the awe and wonder to which this last gives rise. These feelings of the heart give nourishment and life to the will and mind, which, all acting in unison, raise consciousness to a new state of awareness."*

A new state of awareness is soon to arise about cancer, its treatment and prevention. Patients and their loved ones might acknowledge that "meditation is usually made difficult or impossible" trying to understand the disease in the hustle-bustle of a doctor's waiting room or hospital lobby. So in your private moments, make a new commitment to health awareness. Providence will move when you do. Even if all that is changed is your attitude, so that you can confront the specter of cancer less fearfully, you will have achieved a kind of dream vision. Although many people have heard Murray's words about commitment, used as an epigraph to this chapter, few know that he based this insight on this couplet from the German poet Goethe: "Whatever you can do, or dream you can, begin it./Boldness has genius, power, and magic in it."

❧ ❧ ❧

A Lesson of Love from the AIDS Virus

Boston Globe photojournalist Janet Knott says, "In the beginning it wasn't pretty—images of dying men alone in hospital beds—because of a deadly mysterious virus known as AIDS." At the time she took photos of these men in the latter 1980s, the populace feared this disease more than cancer because so little was known about it. "Where did it come from?" she asks, remembering the fearful questions. "Who would get it? Just gay men, or women and children in public restrooms? Could you contract it from blood transfusions or from a visit to the neighborhood dentist?" Years later, in the 21st Century, AIDS still exists but now can be treated. Fear is slowly subsiding with the focus on effective treatment.

Janet remembers a more somber time, photographing what seemed like acres of the AIDS quilt at the mall in Washington, D.C. Janet says it was a lovely spring day. Despite the woven beauty of the AIDS quilt, she notes, the mood was pensive. "In some sense this reminded me of the Viet Nam War Memorial, with visitors quietly paying tribute. But this was different. Unlike the Vietnam War, the battle against AIDS was, and is still, ongoing (although new treatments offer much solace). And the quilt would move from site to site, with the individual quilt of a person who had succumbed to this killer being connected, literally, to a larger community." There is no such quilt for cancer, but nonetheless, we are all bound to fight this battle. To do so, we have to focus on an ally of this enemy associated with the early years of AIDS: *fear*.

That's why we decided to publish Janet's photo of a mother coping with AIDS. "In 1987, Sarah (not her real name) let the me into her life for a year," the photojournalist notes. "Sarah was a mother of three small children and had full-blown AIDS. One day, disgusted with New England weather and weighing just 100 pounds, Sarah boarded a jet and headed for Miami." Soon after her children followed. In the photo in **Figure 14**, Sarah and her then 6-year-old son are enjoying a late afternoon outing at Miami beach. "Love from her children and family was a big reason that Sarah lived as long as she did with this disease," Janet observes. Love also plays a pivotal role in combating cancer. Yes, it lends support and assistance. But it also lessens fear.

"As a photojournalist for 20 years for *The Boston Globe*, I know fear," Janet says. About the same time she took the pictures of dying men alone in hospital beds, she covered the aborted elections in Haiti. "There was much killing," she remembers. "I had to run for my own life then and scale a wall because I feared I might be shot at, too." Love matters in these moments. As Janet tells it, "You want to be comforted instantly by someone who loves you because it makes you feel safe. Strong love has a safety factor to it that overcomes any fear of the future and the unknown." That's a major emphasis of this book.

❦ ❦ ❦

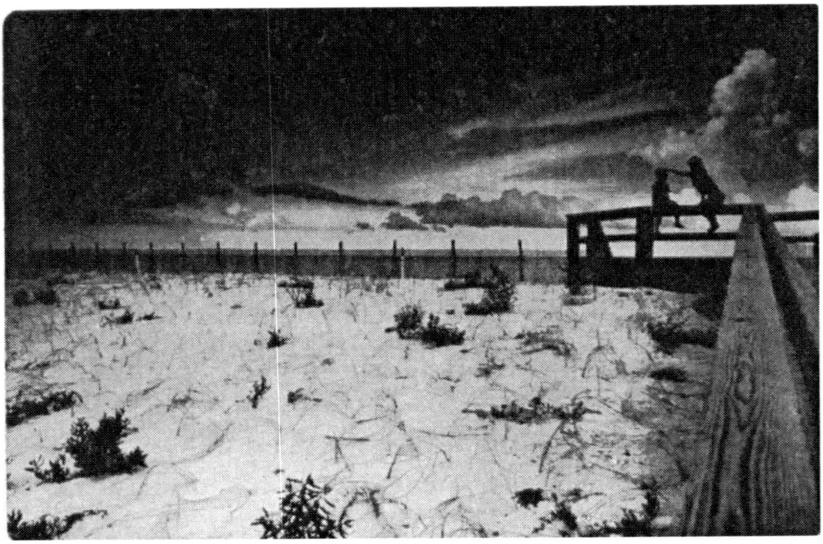

Figure 14.
Sarah and Her Son

Envisioning Exercise

Chronicle Your Commitments to Improve Your Attitude

Objective: To explore commitments you have made that changed your life for the better. This will improve your attitude and aid the healing process.

Physicians increasingly are acknowledging that attitude is a key component during cancer treatment and recovery.

In the "Envisioning Exercise" of the last chapter you noted the high and low points of your life concerning cancer. That helped you get a handle on universal truth and life lessons, increasing your awareness and lessening your fear of cancer. But there is another path to the same destination: recalling "turning points" in your life when you made a commitment—not necessarily associated with illness. (It's the *feeling* of commitment we're trying to evoke, rather than the memory of well being.) You could have made a commitment to another person, for example, as in a marriage or even during childbirth. You could have committed to education, perhaps by enrolling in a university to enhance your mind. Or maybe you wanted to hone your body at a health spa. Or you could have vowed to be gentler or more loving, promising to treat others as you wish to be treated or practicing kindness on a daily basis. Maybe like William Hutchinson Murray you aspired to climb a mountain or write a book.

The types of commitments that people make are as varied as the people making them.

Chronicle your commitments either in your journal, on tape, or in your mind. Ask yourself:

1. What are my turning points, those times when I vowed to commit to an idea or ideal, to a person or practice, to any initiative that ultimately changed my life for the better?

2. What truth or lesson did I learn?

3. How can I resurrect that feeling of commitment so that I can apply the truth or lesson to renewed health?

4. How can I forgive or forget the past disappointments that failed to yield the results that I desired so I can focus on the moment and improve my attitude?

Feel free to share with others your life stories and lessons about commitment.

So much energy is spent regretting fate (especially when you or a loved one is diagnosed with cancer). What better time to remember your golden moments of commitment than now? By doing so you will equip doctors with a new weapon in their growing genetic arsenal: a positive attitude that expands awareness as it enhances the healing process.

Chapter Six

Traditional Therapy

Nothing in life is to be feared. It is only to be understood.
—Madame Curie (1867-1934)

The Earth, you and I are composed of . . . atoms that were created in red giant stars long ago. We are made of starstuff.
—Carl Sagan (1934-1996)

The media play an important role in shaping lay perceptions about science and health care. The media are partly to blame for the general lack of knowledge about the cellular landscape—one of the reasons we decided to write this book. We know that reporters are rarely trained in science and often do not know about the latest, groundbreaking research. Moreover, scientists and physicians explaining cancer treatment often contribute to the problem when they use the jargon of the laboratory rather than the plain speech of the hospital lobby. It should come as no surprise that the most innovative treatments are described in biotechnical and medical journals that few people, even scientists, subscribe to and/or understand.

Here is what usually happens:

1. *The more specialized a discipline like biology or chemistry becomes, the more technical its language becomes.* As new disciplines such as biotechnology and immunology formulate new terms to define concepts or discoveries, new technical languages evolve.

2. *The more technical the language becomes, the fewer the people who understand it.* As each new technolanguage is mastered by members of a discipline, they can discuss key new concepts and discoveries with greater precision (although the best minds of one discipline—say, physics—no longer can easily share ideas with the best minds of another discipline; say, geology). Moreover, fewer lay people understand the new ideas (or even know that they exist).

3. *When researchers and scholars abandon the masses, the popular media fulfill the latter's needs.* As important disciplines relate to fewer and fewer people, specific cultural needs arise within the populace and are satisfied by mass media (especially television). These outlets tend to sensationalize topics, including cancer, needlessly frightening the audience or depicting treatments in stereotypical terms.

4. *The more sensational the media become, the more comfortable the technical disciplines become.* Relieved of the responsibility to share concepts about their disciplines, researchers and physicians sometimes distance themselves from the people they hope to treat, troubled by stereotypical coverage but unaware that they helped create the need for it.

Sensationalism also undermines the value of meditation and spiritual belief and, by extension, *positive attitude*. As we have stated here since the introduction, willing attitudes are *winning* attitudes when it comes to health care. But religion and medicine are being trivialized in the media. Since the late 1980s, for instance, televangelist "healings"—broadcasts about spontaneous recoveries of so-called "true believers"—continue to be popular, with a recent secular twist: *psychic readings*. Your individual spiritualist will explain everything at $5 per minute charged to your phone bill—from your love interest to your health outlook for the coming year . . . or the rest of your life! Worse, even God has gone pop in the wake of the Heaven's Gate tragedy in March 1997. This was one of the tabloid tragedies of the 1990s and played out on the worldwide web in the wake of an awesome cosmological event—the discovery of the Hale-Bopp comet. This celestial wonder should have inspired enlightened discussion about astronomy, about atonement with the universe, about magnificence of creation; instead, the comet faded in the media glare of Heaven's Gate with the mass suicide of 39 cultists.

> **❖ Inspiration Point**
>
> **Readers ought to be in awe in this era as science confirms—bit by bit, byte by byte—cosmological and biological models suggesting a unified design grander than any researcher or theologian might have envisioned.**

Some philosophers say the media factor has cheapened spirituality in our time. The populace ought to be in awe in this era as science confirms—bit by bit, byte by byte—cosmological and biological models suggesting a unified design grander than any researcher or theologian might have envisioned. No one knows what (or if you are religious, who) established natural laws able to spawn a universe out of pinpoint singularity or reverse time at the cellular level via the cloning of a sheep. But the rapturous amazement remains one of the media's yet-to-be told stories.

Instead of watching a television show, gaze outdoors at the night sky. You may be surprised to learn that most scientists believe that Earth is only one of a plentiful number of planets harboring intelligent beings, based on the immense size of the universe and the apparent uniformity of physical laws. This is not a new idea. The prospect of abundant alien life was first discussed during a 1960 conference of physicists and astronomers during which Frank Drake introduced a mathematical model that theorized about a million extraterrestrial civilizations scattered across the Milky Way Galaxy. The late great astronomer Carl Sagan popularized this view in an episode of his PBS series and in a chapter of his accompanying book *Cosmos*. If only 1 percent of civilizations could survive the discovery of atomic bombs, Sagan believed, then the number of existing civilizations in the Galaxy would be in the millions.

Aliens and human beings would not only share atomic bombs and the same galaxy, scientists speculate, they may also share the molecules of life. These molecules will have two things in common: they will have emanated from the solar engine of a star and undergone a mysterious chemical process enabling otherwise inert matter to animate, or come alive. In this chapter we'll take a closer look at those molecules and how they are affected by light and chemistry to help explain the basics of traditional therapies, using simple language and correcting media stereotypes.

❧ ❧ ❧

Images of Traditional Treatment

In most hospitals and cancer centers across the country, cancer treatment consists solely of surgery, radiation therapy, chemotherapy . . . or some combination of these three stalwarts of oncology. Rationale for surgical removal of tumors is obvious. You find a tumor, you excise the tumor. But the logic behind use of radiation therapy and chemotherapy is murkier because of their origins, histories, and media reputations. In part, the media play a role in how we view these treatments. No other image of cancer is more widespread than the picture of a woman or a child devoid of beautiful hair. True, many patients who lose their hair grow it back during recovery or remission. However, photos of recovering cancer patients are largely missing from magazines, newspapers, and television news.

Photos of bald women affect us emotionally. Such images symbolize shame, persecution, and pain the world over. For instance, authorities in some countries still shave the heads of writers to humiliate them. Since ancient times women have had their hair shorn for offenses as petty as not wearing veils in public. And who can forget those haunting pictures of Jewish women who suffered during the Holocaust? Or of bald-headed children worldwide dying not of cancer but of starvation?

Other negative media images are associated with radiation and chemotherapy. Radiation is symbolized by atomic bombs dropped on Hiroshima and Nagasaki. Chemicals are associated with toxic waste, environmental hazards, and pollution. Images that stereotype people affect everyone, and they are disseminated daily to the reading and viewing public. There is a consequence for this. If the public does not have access to health care information described plainly without jargon, it is over-influenced by media coverage. When it comes to cancer, this can be costly, not only with respect to positive attitudes but also in the delaying of treatment. Given this situation, it is increasingly difficult to discuss radiation treatment and chemotherapy rationally.

That's why we delayed this discussion until now. Typically a book about cancer research would begin with traditional therapies and then distinguish old approaches from innovative ones. But we realized the fear factor associated with radiation treatment and chemotherapy, which share a common goal with surgical intervention: *killing cancer*. Surgery kills tumors or parts of tumors by excision. Radiation and chemotherapy try to do the same by killing cells

❖ Inspiration Point

Molecules and families are not only composed of the same starstuff—atoms form molecules for the same motivations as people form families. In a real sense, both seek peace, security, and stability.

that comprise the tumor. In fact, the development of these latter approaches was based solely on random testing of agents to determine their ability to "kill" cancer cells. However, because of this important early research, which has saved tens of thousands of lives, an unfortunate legacy of destructive "killing" agents has emerged. True, the molecular mechanisms by which these agents attack tumor cells were not well understood—initially, at least—even by scientists. But now geneticists see the molecular logic behind their use. This logic may have arrived too late to improve the public's near-term image of radiation treatment and chemotherapy. Nonetheless, researchers and physicians need these therapies in their arsenal against cancer because, when used appropriately, they can be effective, especially when combined with other treatments.

❧ ❧ ❧

Understanding Radiation Treatment

What happens to a tumor when high intensity ionizing radiation is focused on a mass somewhere deep within the body of a cancer patient? Again the answer is found at the molecular level. Diseases that cannot always be effectively treated and/or cured usually have roots at the molecular level. To treat a molecular disease, you have to envision its *progression* during the therapeutic process. So rather than looking at radiation as a "killing" agent aimed at a cancerous mass, you should try to understand both radiation treatment and chemotherapy in the same terms that you have come to understand cancer in the previous chapters of this book, as a *cellular vision*. This, along with the envisioning exercises in this book, can help you overcome the media and medical stereotypes associated with these treatments.

Molecules, of course, are made of connected atoms. Atoms are made up of tinier elements, one of them being an electron, a nearly massless entity with a negative electric charge. Basically, only a limited number of people trained in chemistry know how atomic units of a molecule are held together and why and how they function. However, you don't need to understand this or subatomic physics to appreciate the value of radiation treatment. But it will be helpful to understand fundamental concepts about the inner workings of atomic relationships, especially within the molecules of life.

Remember that an electron is a charged particle. Simply put, when atoms share some of their electrons among each other, instead of keeping them to themselves, electrostatic forces—a bit like the forces between a magnet and an iron object—pull these "electron sharing" atoms together. Atoms that can share electrons in this fashion, and thereby form bonds between themselves, can assemble into molecules. Molecules seem magical because they give us, and everything in the world, shape and dimension. They bestow form. All the molecules of our world, including the molecules of life, are held together by the force of such bonds. When atoms assemble and share electrons, the energy within them is lowered and they become more stable.

In this regard, atoms are a lot like people. A molecule forms in the first place to become a more stable and less "energetic" entity. Consider the "nuclear" family and the close bonds within it. Individuals living alone during the early portion of their adult life often lead very active lives seemingly charged with endless energy, but with marriage and the establishment of family bonds, their lives (theoretically, at least!) become more peaceful, secure, and stable. So molecules and families are not only composed of the same starstuff, atoms form molecules for the same motivations as people form families.

Now that we have demystified atoms somewhat, let's proceed to radiation. The ionizing radiation used in cancer radiation therapy is a form of energy, the most common of which is light. Light and radiation are the same except that ionizing radiation is of much higher potency. Because we are all more familiar with light than radiation, we'll begin by discussing how light interacts with molecules. Then we'll extrapolate this information to ionizing radiation.

Anyone who has ever worn sunglasses or used sunscreen knows that certain materials can absorb light. While natural sunlight contains both visible light and ultraviolet light, only the visible light passes through sunglasses and sunscreen. The ultraviolet light is absorbed by molecules within lenses of the sunglasses or by the chemical molecules in the sunscreen. What happens to the energy of the ultraviolet light? It is present in the rays before it passes through these molecules . . . but is missing when it emerges from them. The answer is because energy cannot be destroyed, only transferred; the ultraviolet light is transferred to and absorbed by the molecules in the sunglass lenses and sunscreen.

These energy-laden molecules become "excited." Ionizing radiation, however, transfers much more energy to energy absorbing molecules than natural light. These molecules become much more excited. This is the intended effect upon which radiation treatment is based. The added energy is transferred into the molecules' electrons, whose nature suddenly changes. In many ways, it's like a divorce. These energetic electrons actually break away from the lower energy situation of "sharing" between an atom and its neighbor to the higher energy situation of "going it alone" as a separate atom again. In effect, ionizing radiation breaks the bonds between atoms.

So molecules, like people, respond in a variety of ways when they acquire excess energy from absorbed light or radiation. This is similar to a stable family that experiences a sudden disruptive force from the outside. Sometimes such a family breaks apart, but often the "charged" situation just results in anger that releases immediate energy so that the family can stabilize again. The same goes for molecules. Some molecules simply release excess energy from light or radiation and come back together again.

We know all about the phenomenon, called *fluorescence,* which helps to illuminate our homes, schools and offices using fluorescent lights. These lights generate fluorescence by a spontaneous release of excess absorbed energy by certain molecules. While some molecules release excess energy as light, other molecules, in different situations, can release energy as heat, for instance. Thus, knowing how molecules release energy is as essential as knowing how they absorb it, for effective radiation treatment.

The size of molecules also matters. Small molecules with no defects in their molecular structure usually release excess energy acquired by the absorption of radiation. They do not break apart. Large polymer molecules and especially DNA usually cannot release this excess energy, but break apart into fragments. This happens for two reasons. First, DNA molecules share electrons in a "smeared" fashion. In other words, there is so much sharing going on that the electrons seem like trees in a forest with branches connecting in a complex molecular network. Because of the smeared sharing of electrons all along the DNA molecule, the excess energy can travel throughout the entire length of the incredibly long molecule. You'll remember from the third chapter that the twisted double helix of DNA, if stretched to full length, is several millimeters long . . . yet only 0.0000020 millimeters wide. That's a dramatic length-to-width ratio. The ratio and folded pattern cause physical stress and local weakness at points along the DNA molecule, creating defects. So when excess energy is absorbed, it prompts the breakage of molecular bonds. For these reasons DNA is unusually susceptible to breakage as a result of the absorption of high-energy radiation.

We already know the consequence of too many breaks within the DNA molecule of a cell. Think again about the gatekeeper suppressor, otherwise known as the "p53" protein. In the presence of such DNA damage, the suppressor triggers the cell-death program. Cells exposed to ionizing radiation experience extensive DNA breakage and are destroyed by the cell-death program. But the issue now is how, if at all, does such radiation therapy distinguish between healthy cells of the body and cancer cells of the tumor?

First of all, radiation in cancer therapy is focused as much as possible upon the tumor so as to maximize the irradiation of cancer cells and to minimize the irradiation of any other cells. But there is another important feature of the cancer cell that we have already discussed, making them much more susceptible to irradiation than normal cells. You'll remember that cancer cells have a short period of time between the cycles of cell division. That's bad news when it comes to DNA repair, but good news when it comes to radiation therapy. Cancer cells may spread quickly but often contain mutations in important DNA repair proteins. That makes the probability of repair from radiation damage much lower in cancer cells than in normal cells. So radiation therapists not only must know how molecules behave when absorbing energy, but how cancer cells do, too. So when it comes to radiation therapy, the tendencies of accumulating mutations—quick replication and poor DNA repair—generally work against the cancer cell and in favor of the healthy cell.

If that were solely the case, however, even advanced stages of cancer would be treatable. Unfortunately, many tumors resist radiation therapy; so sometimes radiation treatment has little or no effect upon the growth of tumors. How can a cell be impervious to powerful irradiation? The idea alone seems absurd, like people being "resistant" to nuclear warfare, which is what radiation therapy actually is at the cellular level. Nonetheless, cancers can be invulnerable to radiation because of mutations in the important "p53" suppressor protein. In effect, without this all-important gatekeeper, cells of the tumor are not slated for death, even in the wake of radiation-induced DNA damage. As you know by now, a mutation in the suppressor protein is the most common mutation found in human cancers, often limiting the usefulness of radiation therapy.

> **❖ Inspiration Point**
>
> **DNA analysis is so important before treatment because the common mutations in a tumor can be monitored. Patients who receive such analyses at therapy centers learn in advance that radiation treatment would be useless if their tumors contain mutations in the "p53" suppressor.**

That's why DNA analysis is so important before treatment—because you can monitor the common mutations in a tumor. Patients who receive such analyses at therapy centers are lucky because they learn in advance that radiation treatment would be useless if their tumors contain mutations in the "p53" suppressor. Not only are they able to forego the side-effects associated with radiation treatment—including fatigue, upset stomach, and skin irritation (depending on the cancer and location of the treatment)—but they are also able to proceed without delay to alternative therapies, including chemotherapy.

❧ ❧ ❧

Understanding Chemotherapy

Chemotherapy can be highly effective against certain malignancies. And while chemotherapy on the surface may seem markedly different from radiation therapy, it is surprisingly similar. The goal is the same: cellular damage by causing a break in DNA, resulting in molecules not sharing electrons, and going it on their own, splitting up, and alerting the ever-ready suppressor protein to respond in great numbers to kill the damaged cells. In fact, most of the chemical agents used in chemotherapy react with the DNA molecule to severely damage it. Some chemotherapeutic drugs actually cleave the DNA molecule and fragment the DNA directly while others chemically modify the DNA in such a way to degrade and break it, halting any repair attempts by the cell. As in radiation therapy, the chemically induced DNA damage also invokes activation of the cell-death program, again via the gatekeeper known as the "p53" suppressor.

However, chemotherapy is unfortunately often not an alternative for a patient with a radiation-resistant tumor. These patients usually lack functional suppressor proteins, rendering the cell-death program useless within their tumors. Cancer cells just go on living even when their DNA has been severely damaged by chemotherapeutic drugs. While the mode of action of most such drugs is similar to that of radiation therapy, because of other aspects of the treatment, chemotherapy has significant differences from radiation therapy.

Chemotherapy shares some side effects with radiation therapy, such as fatigue. It also can cause nausea, vomiting, and hair loss. However, unlike radiation, which can be targeted at a tumor, chemotherapy is administered to the body as a whole. The side effects have little to do with the chemical agents' ability to seek out cancerous cells. In this regard, chemotherapy can be even more effective than radiation therapy because the chemical substances are carried by body fluids to the more rapidly dividing cells. Moreover, the most highly effective chemotherapeutic drugs were discovered by screening many substances known to react with DNA to see which ones best selected tumor cells.

Because of such random testing, researchers do not always know the mechanisms of chemical agents that target tumor cells. The targeting of such cells is called "selectivity." If researchers fully understood these mechanisms, perhaps chemotherapy would be more effective, as new classes of drugs could be manufactured. Every day there is hope that this traditional therapy will become even more effective in the future. In general, though, the basis for selectivity of chemical agents is the rate of division of their intended target cells. To envision this, think of "target" practice. The chemical "agent" like an FBI officer sits on a rapidly moving Jeep through the cellular terrain, firing at the moving targets of cancer cells. With the agent and the target in motion, misfires can occur. After all, chemotherapeutic drugs aim at rapidly dividing cells and so suffer the same drawbacks. That's why chemotherapy is often lethal to non-cancerous cells that naturally divide at an accelerated rate. In effect, it mistakes rapidly dividing healthy cells for typically fast-replicating cancerous cells. Healthy cells that divide rapidly include those within hair follicles.

Hair-follicle cells continually divide to allow for continued growth of hair. Because they have a high rate of turnover, they become targets for many chemotherapeutic drugs. That's why hair loss is often associated with chemotherapy. As we've discussed earlier, the cells on the surface of the intestine, as well as the remainder of the digestive tract, have a high turnover rate. For this reason, loss of some digestive functions also is associated with chemotherapy.

❖ Inspiration Point

Traditional therapies and their basic components—light and chemistry, the elements of life—can restore life when used appropriately against cancer.

Most chemotherapeutic drugs target the tumor cell's DNA. But a few newer drugs act by another mechanism and destroy rapidly dividing cells by disrupting a different aspect of the cell's machinery. These drugs, the most well known of which is Taxol, disrupt the cellular machinery that actually divides the cell from one entity into two. They do not target DNA and do not apparently activate the cell-death program through the suppressor protein "p53." As you can see, such drugs may prove especially useful in patients with cancers containing mutations in this vital gatekeeper. In addition to the chemotherapeutic drugs discussed here are several that do not simply "kill" tumor cells, but inhibit certain pathways involved in the formation or promotion of specific tumors. These are an important class of drugs in the struggle against cancer which we will discuss later.

For the moment, think about the cellular strategies of these traditional therapies and their basic components—light and chemistry, the elements of life—and how both can restore life when used appropriately against cancer. And ponder the wisdom of Marie Curie, the Nobel-winning physicist-chemist who discovered radium, which paved the way for radiation treatment: *"Nothing in life is to be feared. It is only to be understood."* Madame Curie, whose courage has inspired generations, also said: *"I never see what has been done; I only see what remains to be done."*

❧ ❧ ❧

The Concept of Discretion

The ethical concept of discretion has a key component: *time*. Discretion implies time because it sets priorities. You spend an hour watching a television show rather than doing a chore, rather than paying a bill. We make daily decisions about time and how we will spend it.

Illness, or the prevention thereof, traditionally is a great setter of priorities. You learn that life is precious not because of professional ambition or personal happiness but because of time, a limited amount, otherwise called *your life*. You are born at one point in time and will end at another point in time. There is good evidence—some scientific, some philosophical—that nature develops consciousness for a reason beyond our immediate grasp. As any biologist will tell you, birth and death are natural and fundamental to time. It's one of nature's laws that even applies to cells in the body. Philosophers also know that illness reminds us about boundaries, some related to time and others related to importance. Consider the old saying: *no one approaching the end of life complains about not spending enough time at the office*. In the end, illness reminds us of the things that are timeless within all of us: the meaning of life, the meaningfulness of love.

Illness is also a quick teacher of discretion. With whom should you share information about your medical condition? Your symptoms? Side effects? Discretion also involves learning. What information should you allow into your psyche and what to block out? What to question? What to embrace?

The media associate illness with *lack* of time, the stereotypical image of an hour glass whose sands slowly run out, along with your dreams. But in actuality, illness slows pace even as it teaches about discretion and priorities. Illness changes daily routine. Jobs or tasks sometimes come to a halt. You also spend a lot of time waiting—for the next doctor, for the next diagnosis, for the next drug.

The problem is that free time emanating out of illness often is accompanied by fear. Fear of firing if an employer knows about illness or symptoms. Fear of financial loss if insurance is insufficient or non-existent. Fear of the doctor, the diagnosis, the drug. Fear of lack of fulfillment. So many phobias can arise with respect to cancer that so little time is left to do anything else *but* fear.

Fear of time running out. We then replay those same fears over and over, undermining the positive attitude that enhances wellness.

To undermine fear and enhance wellness, remember the words of astronomer Carl Sagan: "you are starstuff." You are *more* than starstuff. You are *smart* starstuff. Your mind is as expansive as the universe. So much so that you can befriend a star. Possess it. Go out on the deck or to the window and claim a star simply by choosing one in the sky. After all, light is there for the taking. No one owns the stars except for those who behold them. And there's mystery in the choosing. That star on the outer edges of the galaxy may not be a star at all but a distant galaxy so far away that clusters of billions of stars only seem like one star on the horizon. See what you can possess through your consciousness? If you look at that star or galaxy long enough, you'll know it's there even when the clouds obscure it. You will have absorbed it via your mind and memory. That star or galaxy is light, and light triggers chemical reactions, as you have learned in this chapter. But some ethicists and many artists also believe that a metaphoric light exists in each of us and, when our consciousness expands enough, we are guided by that light—as sailors are guided by stars—even in our darkest hours.

To hearken the light within you, lose yourself in the timeless nature of art, especially music. Compose some if you can, or else listen to your favorite opera or melody and immerse yourself in memory or meditation. Shut off the television, especially the nightly news, with its myriad stories of horror, war, lies, oppression, and mean-spirited politics. You always have time for that. You always can find it at any hour on cable. Practice discretion when it comes to media consumption because fear is programmed in the news, even weather coverage. A report about a hurricane, flood, or tornado also implies: *This can happen to you.* Today, though, you have set some priorities. Not only are you going to own a star and a song but also envision how you will live the rest of your life, no matter how long or how short, in the timelessness of the moment.

❦ ❦ ❦

Envisioning Exercise

Enhance Relationships

Objective: To focus on enhancing your relationships and to push out worry and fear from your mind.

To do this exercise, meditate or write in your journal about the following:

1. The meaningfulness of your relationships with a family member, a child, a friend, or significant other. What common bonds did or do you share with these people that either inspired or somehow uplifted you? What issues, if any, have come between you that still continue unresolved?

2. If you had one year left with each person, what feelings would you nurture? What disagreements would you resolve? What would you do with this person—take a trip? attend an event? celebrate, however belatedly, an accomplishment?

3. If you only had fifteen minutes of time remaining with each person, what would you say to reaffirm your relationship or to heal a rift?

4. Do the exercise again from the *other* person's perspective. How would that person answer each question posed in numbers 1-3 above?

5. If that person is available, and the situation is appropriate and loving, ask him or her to do exercises 1-3 above and then compare *(a)* your response, *(b)* the response you imagined the person would proffer, and *(c)* that person's actual response.

6. Meditate or write about the similarities and differences in responses *a, b,* and *c* above.

Doing the envisioning exercises above will not only expand your consciousness but also your perception and priorities. Use your free time—not to worry or fear—but to enhance your relationships that shape and give meaning to your life.

Chapter Seven

Gene Therapy: A Great Yet Limited Hope

Just as the proverbial forest is hidden by its trees, the tree of life itself is hidden by its luxurious canopy.
—Christian de Duve (1917-)

Anybody who has been seriously engaged in scientific work of any kind realizes that over the entrance to the gates of the temple of science are written the words: Ye must have faith. It is a quality which the scientist cannot dispense with.
—Max Planck (1858-1947)

Basics of Gene Therapy

By now you know two vital bits of information about cancer:

- *Mutations spawn defects in genes that control the cell cycle.*
- *Additional mutations cause defects in the body's natural safeguards, allowing the uncontrolled expansion of cancer cells.*

Perhaps you also are beginning to recognize how cancer differs from other diseases. Certainly it is distinct in both its origins and progression from diseases caused by invaders like bacteria and viruses, which can be cured simply by destroying these foreign assailants. Although the onset of cancer can be triggered by outside elements or lifestyles—primarily smoking, poor diet, lack of exercise, and obesity—cancer really is the result of *an accumulation of defects within our own system.* In other words, your body manufactures the cancer. Tumor cells are the patient's very own cells that differ from normal ones only in tiny specific changes in a handful of their thousands of genes. That's why mutations master stealth, often eluding detection by the body's own defense mechanisms.

For this reason, traditional means of cancer treatment, including radiation and chemotherapy, may be only marginally effective. As mentioned in the previous chapter, even highly sophisticated and effective present day anti-tumor drugs kill normal cells—including ones of the digestive lining and hair follicles—almost as fast as they kill targeted tumor cells.

> **❖ Inspiration Point**
>
> **A basic change in attitude—restoring the cell via new therapies instead of killing it via traditional ones—may lead sooner rather than later to a cure for various cancers.**

Cancer also differs from heart disease, the nation's top killer. Heart and other degenerative diseases involve malfunction of action molecules—ones that replenish the muscle proteins, for instance. This can cause the heart muscle to weaken so that the organ cannot constrict enough to pump sufficient blood. Cancer, on the other hand, is the result of direct damage to the genes themselves. This involves DNA, the most basic molecule of life. With each chapter you have been learning more about the miraculous complexity of this molecule and its supporting cast: a host of vital proteins, especially the gatekeepers, as archetypal as archangels at the four gates of Eden. Geneticists may admire the complexity and archetype of DNA, but they also know the challenge that awaits them. The intricate features of DNA demand intricate means and methods to treat cancer. The good news is that medical scientists are acquiring reliable information about the functions of genes and proteins operating as the molecules of life. Computer technology will continue to develop, allowing scientists to map the cellular landscape with startling pre-

❖ Inspiration Point

Biologically, we all share the same ancient mother, known as "Mitochondrial Eve." Our DNA may be complex, but it is also common. Complexity is the challenge, commonality, the hope for a cure.

cision. Knowledge, fear's enemy, doubles worldwide every 20 or so months—thanks to communication technology. Databases are updated daily. On the whole, we are especially optimistic about medical science's meeting the challenges of cancer, especially via gene therapy. In many ways, determining how to treat the disease will *define* medicine in the 21st Century, since most of the challenges facing medicine now have their origins within the deepest and most basic molecule of life.

❧ ❧ ❧

An Exciting, New Approach

DNA has a luxurious canopy, countless microscopic stems and branches upon which thousands of genes like Edenic fruit hang from our common Tree of Life. On that tree is the name "Eve" inscribed on the cell's mitochondria (pronounced *"MITE-oh-CON-dree-ah")*, a kind of cellular fuel refinery, allowing reactions to occur within and between cells. Eve, or as biologists prefer, "Mitochondrial Eve," probably lived some 200,000 years ago in Africa, passing along a key trait in our DNA that led humans up the evolutionary ladder. Not only is our DNA complex, but also common. The complexity is the challenge, but the commonality is the hope. For if scientists can peer under the canopy long enough, they might find the right pathways to treat or cure all cancers. And those therapies, whatever their number or complexity, would apply to us all . . . because we all share the molecules of life.

> **❖ Inspiration Point**
>
> **Repairing cells via gene therapy—rather than removing tumors or killing cancerous cells via traditional chemotherapy and radiation—is a *simple, elegant* idea . . . meeting basic requirements of scientific truth.**

Gene therapy not only requires a cellular vision but also faith in a new approach to treatment. This approach, as it applies to cancer and other diseases, lies not in destroying aberrant tissue—i.e. surgically removing tumors or using radiation and chemotherapy to kill tumor cells. The answer may be in *repairing* the molecules of life. Why not? Since the aberrant cells of cancerous tissue are obeying the faulty commands of their DNA, a medical team should heal the tissue by repairing its DNA. The idea is both elegant and simple, two requirements of scientific truth. That notion comes down to us in part from William of Occam, a 13th Century English cleric and philosopher, who is credited with a statement now regarded as one of the turning points in the biological sciences, Occam's Razor, which reads: "*plurality should not be assumed without necessity*." Or in modern lingo, "*Keep it simple*." That notion, fundamentally, helped bring medieval science out of the dark ages and into the modern realm. Likewise geneticists now believe that repairing DNA rather than destroying tumor cells may be the simple, elegant answer to cancer that has been eluding us all along.

The first faint gleaming of this answer appeared on the horizon in the 1970s when scientists first learned how to introduce new genes into laboratory mice. This breakthrough, and studies emanating out of it, clearly demonstrated that a supply of "correct" genes could supplement the function of faulty ones resulting from mutations. With this knowledge medical scientists began to imagine treating genetic damage and DNA mutations by "doctoring" the DNA itself. This new therapeutic concept became known as "gene therapy." This dream is already a reality as new gene therapy protocols (treatment plans) have entered clinics and are just now beginning to be used to address a variety of diseases, including cancer. To understand gene therapy, we need to explore a bit more about ground-breaking studies in this discipline.

❧ ❧ ❧

An Overview of Therapies

Early attempts at mastering gene therapy frustrated researchers. These scientists were experimenting on mice, using the smallest imaginable needle to accomplish the first gene transfer: injecting tiny amounts of man-made DNA fragments, containing new genes, into the nucleus of just fertilized eggs. Within this realm of the chromosomes, the DNA repair mechanisms took over. They spliced the added DNA fragments into chromosomal breaks, the way a construction crew might fill potholes on the cellular terrain. All this took place inside the egg, the one cell from which all the other cells of the newly formed mouse would be fashioned. And it worked. Scientists had succeeded in transferring genes into a living animal. But they were also frustrated by the fact that the *means* they used to place genes into the chromosomes of laboratory animals could never be used in human genetic therapy. Since the transfer of the added genes needed to be done within a fertilized egg, a physician would have to learn within hours of the conception of his patient that he or she would someday need genetic treatment. Furthermore, this clairvoyant physician would also have to somehow know the exact genetic defect this child would develop. Clearly, researchers realized, other methods would have to be developed to add "therapeutic genes" to the cells of diseased tissue in adult patients.

> **❖ Inspiration Point**
>
> **Biologists always ask themselves how something they wish to accomplish is done in nature. Then, they employ nature or mimic it to serve a missing function or desired end. That type of thinking has helped advance gene therapy.**

Motivated by this challenge, researchers had faith that they would develop effective strategies. A dedicated group of molecular biologists, geneticists and physicians confronted—and resolved—the first problem: finding some means of getting the therapeutic DNA to and into the billions of target cells of a patient's body. This might seem like an impossible task unless you begin to think like a biologist. Physicists, especially cosmologists, think like philosophers and are moved more by the beauty than the simplicity of an idea. Mathematicians, like accountants, value precision along with beauty and simplicity. But biologists always ask themselves how something they wish to accomplish is done in nature. Once they determine this, they employ nature or mimic it to serve a missing function or desired end. So biologists pondered natural methods to effectively introduce DNA into the cells of a person.

In this regard, nature can teach us a lot. We all have extensive experience with the agents that introduce material into our cellular makeup. Viruses, for instance, are little more than a package of DNA wrapped within an effective delivery vehicle. Once a viral DNA has been delivered to the infected cell it encodes its viral proteins and begins to manufacture its offspring viruses using your cellular machinery to do its job. You, of course, become sick because this misuse of your cells damages or destroys them. And yet, if viruses can deliver viral DNA for their usual evil purpose, why not the useful DNA of therapeutic genes for a good purpose? Again, the idea was elegant and simple. So when researchers asked themselves this question, they responded with a resonant, "Why not?"

> **❖ Inspiration Point**
>
> **Since nature evolved clever viruses to deliver DNA to our cells, why not use them to safely deliver a *therapeutic cargo* to diseased cells?**

In some of the earliest examples of true genetic engineering, these researchers literally rebuilt the package. They manufactured viruses devoid of their payload of viral DNA, carrying therapeutic genes instead. The earliest type of virus used as vehicles to deliver therapeutic genes were retroviruses, the type that includes the HIV virus that causes AIDS. More recently, researchers have effectively used adenoviruses (pronounced *"ADD-no-VIGH-rus-es"*), typically found in mild respiratory infections. But none of these vehicles carry much danger since they contain only the outer trappings of the virus and are without its dangerous viral genes. Furthermore, without their viral genes, these man-made vehicles for DNA delivery cannot replicate and spread through generation after generation of infections. In fact, once these vehicles have delivered their curative DNA to diseased cells, their mission and their life span is over. These man-made "viruses" are just "one round fighters" in the bout against disease. What if treatment required not a first-round knockout but a technical one over many rounds in the cellular ring? Scientists again looked to nature for an answer. Since nature evolved clever viruses to deliver DNA to our cells, why not use them to safely deliver a *therapeutic cargo* to diseased cells?

Researchers soon found other delivery systems as efficient as therapeutic viruses, giving more options to physicians who wish to use gene therapy. In the 21st Century, the age of gene therapy is upon us with all of its hope and promise to fight diseases of DNA with therapy of that same DNA. In the late 1990s, gene therapy protocols were not yet generally available to patients with cancer. But numerous clinical trials on a few selected cancer patients have been in progress across the United States in many cancer treatment centers. Moreover, a limited number of these protocols already have advanced beyond the trial stage and are now being used generally at a few specialized centers. Certainly, the age of cancer gene therapy has begun. But exactly how is gene therapy being used to treat cancer?

❧ ❧ ❧

Overcoming the Limitations

Back to that all-important gatekeeper protein known by its "p53"-atomic weight (the suppressor). We already know that mutations in this gatekeeper are associated with the initiation or the progression of many cancers. Also, we learned in the previous chapter, that when the suppressor ceases to function properly, a tumor becomes resistant to radiation and most forms of chemotherapy. So patients having tumors with this mutation have the least chance of effective treatment by conventional means. Since mutations here render the "p53" protein non-functional, the suppressor cannot trigger programmed cell death in response to extensive DNA damage caused by radiation or chemotherapy. So, why not simply add a new "p53" gatekeeper gene to these cancer cells, revitalizing these lost functions?

Researchers are trying to do just that. Several very promising clinical trials using engineered viral vehicles carrying a suppressor gene are in progress. One of these trials targeted patients with the dreaded "small cell" lung carcinoma containing mutations in the suppressor gene. Since patients with this cancer presently have no effective therapy, this new experimental gene therapy was a last hope for those who volunteered for this trial. The "p53" gene was incorporated into an adenovirus delivery package, made from a respiratory virus we have all probably been infected with many times. These engineered gene therapy viruses were injected into the patient's tumors, and many of those tumors regressed and shrunk substantially. Unfortunately, while the gene therapy prolonged the life of many of those treated, all eventually died of their disease. As is common in the battle against cancer, researchers became frustrated. Why did this conceptually ideal treatment fail to cure the patients who received this gene therapy?

Remember the odious characteristic of all cancer cells. They divide faster then their neighbors and a few such cells can easily expand to generate a tumor. If gene therapy could introduce a corrective gene like the "p53" gatekeeper into 100% of all the cells of a tumor, perhaps gene therapy could truly cure cancer. Unfortunately, no gene therapy vehicle can deliver a therapeutic gene with such perfect efficiency. Most likely, those patients in the gene therapy trial for small cell lung cancer were "cured" of the cell cycle defect in those cancer cells receiving the new "p53" gene. These cells either returned to a less dangerous pre-cancerous state or were destroyed by the natural cell death program. But what of the cancer cells that did not receive the corrective gene? Certainly, they established new cancer foci and re-established the disease within the lungs of these patients. Because even one uncorrected cancer cell can re-establish the disease, gene therapy aimed at replacing lost gene function to cure cancer must be 100% efficient to work. The efficiency of delivering corrective genes to tumor cells is only a little more than 10% for most vehicles used today. This is one of the major limitations of gene therapy. Even viruses, which have evolved over millions of years to efficiently deliver DNA, cannot infect 100% of their target cells. Scientists looking for ways to introduce the "p53" gatekeeper into every cancer cell have an eye on the sign at the temple gates of science: *Ye must have faith.* Nonetheless, it is unlikely that this limitation in gene therapy will be overcome quickly or easily. At the moment gene therapy might be effective in some cases, even though it is inefficient. But there is more hope on the cellular horizon.

❧ ❧ ❧

A New Class of Drugs

One simple approach to a more effective use of gene therapy against cancer might be to treat tumors over and over again. This way, physicians would introduce corrective genes to a greater and greater fraction of their cancer cells, with each successive round gaining on mutations until all the cells of the tumor have been revitalized. That presents another problem, though. While biologists often look to nature to solve problems, sometimes nature gets in the way. For instance, because most of the vehicles used in gene therapy are derived from viruses, which are foreign to our bodies, our immune system quickly responds to these foreign proteins and finally rejects these messengers of hope. But overcoming this limitation may soon be possible as new agents are being developed that can avoid immune rejection.

> **❖ Inspiration Point**
>
> **Luck in the lab is defined by faith—the persistent belief that an idea is right—and the willingness to keep at it while keeping it simple. This mindset is yielding results every day in laboratories nationwide.**

An exciting novel use of gene therapy, which is remarkably effective, combines this new age therapy with chemotherapy. Several decades ago a drug was developed by the pharmaceutical industry to destroy cells infected with Herpes virus and to thus destroy the virus within a patient. This drug is truly a forerunner of a new class of drugs, innocuous to normal cells, but which can be activated by reaction with a foreign protein of the Herpes virus into a chemical as powerful as chemotherapeutic drugs. These drugs have come to be known as "pro-drugs," which require specific activation within their target cells to become deadly. Many people infected with Herpes virus take this pro-drug routinely with virtually no side effects, yet those cells within their bodies that are infected with the Herpes virus are instantly killed.

Cancer researchers took note. They wondered if it might be possible to introduce the Herpes virus gene, which produced the viral protein that was able to activate this powerful pro-drug, into tumor cells. They theorized that if this could be accomplished by gene therapy, the "engineered" tumor cells would then become targets for this powerful pro-drug. Imagine the possibilities! A powerful anti-tumor chemotherapeutic drug would be completely harmless to the other body cells. Cancer patients on effective chemotherapy would not suffer debilitating side effects of their treatment. This, of course, would mean no more media photos of bald cancer patients, weakened not only by their disease but by its treatment. Fear of treatment would decrease, generating better attitudes about cancer. Could such hopes be achieved using gene therapy methods, introducing only the pro-drug activating gene into little more than 10% of the tumor's cancer cells? At first it certainly did not seem so, but sometimes, even in cancer research, good luck is even better than a good idea. And in the lab, luck is defined by faith—the persistent belief that an idea is right—and the willingness to keep at it while keeping it simple. The more persistent the scientist, the greater the odds of lucking out. And that is precisely what happened with this experimental therapy.

When researchers first tried their new idea on laboratory mice with tumors, the results were dramatically successful. Although these scientists showed clearly that they were only able to introduce the activating gene into about 10% of the tumor cells, the entire tumor was destroyed with no side effects to the animal. How could this have happened? Even the sophisticated medical researchers who carried out these experiments had no idea. Within a few years, more information about tumor cells became available on cancer databases nationwide. Finally, a plausible explanation emerged. Because of changes in the surface characteristics of tumor cells resulting from their uncontrolled growth and loss of specialization, tiny bridges form between these malignant cells. These cellular bridges are micro-tubes that allow small molecules to pass freely between and among the cells in a tumor. So while only 10% of the treated tumor cells contained the gene and produced the protein that activated the pro-drug, the now active drug could spread to all of the remaining 90% of the cells of the tumor, destroying them efficiently. This time, cancer's intricate network of quick replication was working against it. Those micro-bridges allowed anti-cancer platoons to cross into new terrain, eliminating the enemy mutations.

The initial results were so promising that this approach was advanced quickly to clinical trials with cancer patients. This occurred because the side effects were negligible, and there already existed several decades of clinical experience with this pro-drug in patients with Herpes virus infections. The first subjects recruited into trials of this revolutionary new therapeutic approach were patients with inoperable brain tumors. As most people are aware, patients with brain tumors often receive a very pessimistic prognosis because there is often no effective therapy. Now, researchers speculated, there might be.

Gene therapy vehicles were loaded with the herpes virus and the pro-drug activating gene and injected into the tumors of these patients. The patients were then given daily doses of the pro-drug for several weeks. The results of these trials were encouraging but not conclusive. But the therapy worked with some brain tumors, meaning an effective treatment for these cancers might soon be at hand. Yet further studies of this new combined gene/drug therapy are needed to perfect this approach. One exciting possibility is that repeated treatments with this therapy may be possible. The immune system is shielded from the region of the brain and so immune rejection, which thwarts repeated use of gene

❖ Inspiration Point

If you are becoming excited about the possibilities of gene therapy, you share that feeling with scientists. Usually skeptical about new treatments, scientists are enthusiastically conducting experiments and clinical trials. *Ideas abound.*

therapy in other tissues, may not block its repeated use at this particular body site. Certainly, this new gene-assisted chemotherapy will help to destroy the image of chemotherapy as a devastating and painful therapy since patients in early trials of this new method experienced no side effects from the drug (**see Figure 15**).

The potential for this gene-therapeutic approach to brain tumors, along with a wide range of other tumors, is tremendously significant. In many ways this approach signals the beginning of a new era in cancer therapy and the promise of effective cancer gene therapy. In addition to pro-drug activation and "p53" gene addition, many other strategies and trials using different approaches and different genes are presently in progress. Cancer researchers are uncharacteristically optimistic about early results from these studies, and this has sparked more research using a wide array of approaches.

For the first time in decades, cancer researchers are motivated by innovation in the treatment of cancer. One of the most exciting ideas does not even involve gene therapy, but evolved from a central aspect of gene therapy research. Scientists studying the adenovirus vehicle used to deliver therapeutic genes learned an interesting and now useful aspect of the means by which the natural virus subverts the cells it infects, so as to allow them to produce more viruses. This is what they deduced: since the infecting virus needs much of the cellular machinery of DNA replication—active during cell division—to replicate the invading virus, the virus must *inactivate* the cellular "p53" suppressor gene. This turns on the cell cycle, and you recall what can occur with an inactive

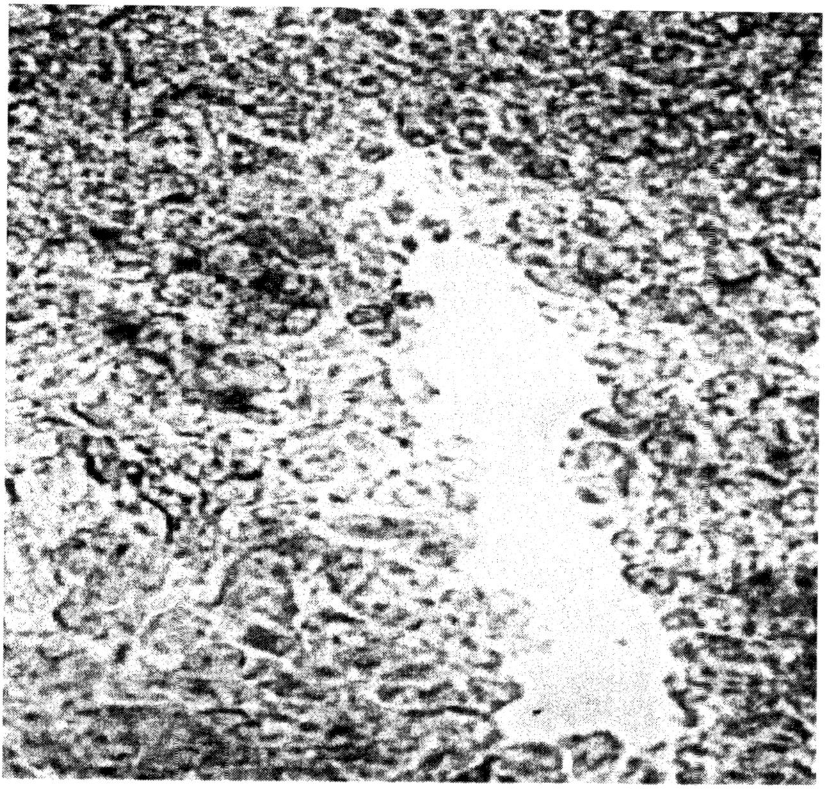

Figure 15.
Gene Therapy: A Cellular Vision

Here gene therapy activates a pro-chemotherapeutic drug to destroy a tumor. Approximately 10 percent of the cells around the needle tract from an injection spread the activated pro-drug to the other tumor cells.

suppressor—the beginnings of cancer. Now this rapidly dividing cell can pump out lots of new viruses, borrowing the cell's replication machinery. You might think a virus that did this would cause cancer, but since the virus eventually destroys the cell it infects, this does not happen. As luck would have it, because the scientists studying this aspect of adenoviruses were trained as cancer researchers, they soon began to devise ways to use this characteristic of adenoviruses as a cancer therapy.

Normal adenoviruses can infect and kill any cell. Scientists analyzing these viruses happened upon a mutant strain of adenovirus. This strain cannot inactivate the "p53" gatekeeper and cannot survive and copy itself in normal cells. Therefore this virus is totally safe to the body's normal cells. But what about a cancer cell that already has a defective, inactive "p53" suppressor protein? This mutant adenovirus can survive and copy itself inside a cancer cell with a "p53" mutation. In effect now, the virus not only kills the cancer cell but reproduces more viruses to kill more such cancer cells, effectively shrinking or even eliminating tumors.

This therapy has a lot going for it. In a sense, it introduces cellular suicide into the mutant landscape. Better yet, the treatment is easily adaptable. The ability to re-engineer this virus was almost commonplace among cancer researchers who spent years modifying it to serve as a gene therapy vehicle. So it was reasonable to imagine altering it in other ways as well. Of course, this modified virus was now completely unable to replicate and survive in normal cells. The tables finally had been turned on the potentially lethal "p53" mutation that you have read about in previous chapters. A mutation in that vital gatekeeper, finally, is no longer a key obstacle in the search for effective treatment. Thus, in a common cancer cell, this specially modified virus could replicate and spread to other such cancer cells, potentially killing them all. We all can recognize the potential of such a cancer-killing virus that cannot infect another of the patient's cells. While clinical trials of this novel therapy for tumor cells with "p53" mutations has just recently begun, it is a promising new treatment for cancers now resistant to most conventional therapies.

Gene therapy and related methods for the treatment of cancer have probably brought more optimism to the community of cancer researchers and physicians than has any other advancement in the history of this disease. As scientists work within the limitations of this powerful new therapeutic approach, many new therapies for the effective treatment of many types of cancer will likely be developed and become widely available within the next decade. But the extent to which these new therapies will change the landscape of oncology and alter the outlook for patients with a cancer diagnosis is yet to be determined.

The good news is that researchers can look under the lush canopy of DNA and devise effective strategies. The ones developed today will be enhanced for patients tomorrow, restoring faith not only in those who enter the temple gates of science but also the revolving doors of cancer clinics.

❧ ❧ ❧

How Much Faith Do You Have?

Faith is an ethical concept associated with hope. Hope is the desire for some future end result—the feeling that despite odds, things will turn out to be in one's favor. It is critical, however, to distinguish between scientific and religious faith. The latter has to do with belief in a supreme being, creator, or afterlife. Ethicists know that this, in essence, cannot be known because of a philosophical concept called "the human condition." Simply put, that means that you, a being of consciousness—connected intimately with the universe and a product of natural law—know that life ends. And yet a feeling lingers that somehow, some way, you will go on eternally. How you handle that conundrum is the focus of every world religion, some with a deity as the focus and some with no deity whatsoever.

Scientific faith, on the other hand, is based on reason. But feelings are involved, too. In the lab, a geneticist theorizes some end result, based on natural law. And when his or her experiment does not conclusively achieve that desired result, a good scientist gets to the bottom of things by being persistent. He or she has faith in natural law. That includes hope, the feeling that any limitation, however seemingly insurmountable, can be overcome in the laboratory. You can see how this applies to gene therapy and to Max Planck's motto of heeding the "faith" motto on the temple gates of science.

How much, and what kind, do *you* have? In some sense it is important for a person seeking to understand, treat or prevent cancer to have both scientific and religious faith. Ethicists believe in a good balance They strive to know the meaning of the human condition and, like scientists, have great respect for natural law. As an example of the importance of having religious faith in addition to scientific faith, there is scientific evidence that religious faith can alleviate depression. For instance, researchers studied a group of the elderly suffering from depression and found that those with religious conviction achieved improvement in the shortest amount of time. In a recent article in *Science News*, one of the researchers—psychiatrist Harold Koenig of Duke University Medical Center—stated: "Religious faith may provide such persons with a sense of hope that things will turn out all right regardless of their problems and thus foster greater motivation to achieve emotional recovery." If you can achieve a level balance of religious and scientific faith, you also may be able to attain a positive attitude *and* an informed opinion. That will help you make sound decisions for yourself and your loved ones.

Envisioning Exercise

Exploring Your Faith and the Meaning of Life

Objective: To better understand your faith and the meaning of your life, enabling you to develop and maintain a more positive attitude.

Before reading ahead, please do the following three-part envisioning exercise in the precise order presented:

I. Accessing Faith

Ask yourself:

- ❖ If I had to assign a percentage, what portion of 100% would I assign to my religious or spiritual faith? What percentage to scientific faith?
- ❖ If I am lacking in one or the other, what can I actively do, and what books can I read to reacquaint myself so as to achieve both an informed opinion and a balance?
- ❖ What ends do I desire and how, precisely, can each type of faith—religious, scientific—help me understand my own and the human condition?

Record your answers in a journal or on a tape machine or ask someone to help you record your answers.

II. Discovering Your Life "Story"

In earlier envisioning exercises you charted the highs, lows, and turning points of your life. Refer to those answers now. String them together in chronological order and "discover" the plot line of your life. Chances are, you will find one, a story of repeating opportunities (or fears) gone unaddressed or unfulfilled until you reached a turning point in your hopes, ambitions, relationships, and/or dreams.

Ask yourself:

- ❖ What knowledge can you take from this life story? What purpose or lesson?
- ❖ What are the common themes, especially ones associated with fear? How, if at all, has knowledge helped ease those fears?
- ❖ What events or opportunities from your youth have presented themselves again later in life? What meaning can you derive from that?

Again, record your answers in a journal or on a tape machine or ask someone to help you do this.

III. Using Occam's Razor

Now let's think like the cleric/scientist William Occam who believed that truth is found in the simplest, most elegant answers. Review your responses to exercises I and II and ponder the simplest, most elegant truths about your life. In those responses you should find the threads of faith, hope, belief, and reason. Use them to develop and maintain a more positive attitude because of renewed balance and enhanced knowledge.

Finally, let's explore the meaning of life. Each person defines that meaning subjectively, including scientists. To help you put this envisioning exercise into perspective, ponder the wise words about the meaning of life from the book *Vital Dust* by Nobel laureate Christian de Duve, who shared the 1974 prize for biology and medicine for his work on the structural and functional organization of the cell:

> "If the universe is not meaningless, what is its meaning? For me, this meaning is to be found in the structure of the universe, which happens to be such as to produce thought by way of life and mind. Thought, in turn, is a faculty whereby the universe can reflect upon itself, discover its own structure, and apprehend such immanent entities as truth, beauty, goodness, and love."

Chapter Eight

❦ ❦ ❦

Immunotherapy: Helping the Body Cure Itself

These germs of disease have taken toll of humanity since the beginning of things—taken toll of our prehuman ancestors since life began here. But by virtue of natural selection of our kind we have developed resisting power; to no germs do we succumb without a struggle. . . . By the toll of a billion deaths man has bought his birthright of the earth, and it is his against all comers. . . . For neither do men live nor die in vain.

—H. G. Wells (1866-1946)

At the turn of the century there was much optimism about the power of the immune system. As early as 1796 scientists knew about the body's ability to ward off disease. That year Edward Jenner injected people with cowpox to protect them from smallpox. But only toward the end of the 19th Century did researchers understand the basic mechanisms at work in the immune system. And yet a novelist popularized the idea in a philosophical book so universal that its truths still resonate today.

H. G. Wells' *The War of the Worlds,* published in 1898, is now considered a science fiction classic. In it are startling images foreboding scientific progress like laser technology and social catastrophes like World War II. The plot concerns an invasion from Mars. High-tech aliens easily destroy human defensive armies until Western civilization seems ready to collapse. Humans prevail, however, in part because of morality and in part because of the immune system. The mighty invaders from Mars have superior weaponry and inferior immune systems, dropping dead on the battlefield not from wounds but from earthly diseases from which humans have been protected for eons.

The War of the Worlds is also famous for another reason: a hoax that spread fear across the United States. In 1938, on the eve of All Saints Day, entertainer Orson Welles broadcast a radio version of H. G. Wells' novel. Welles rewrote the setting for the alien invasion. Instead of landing in England, the Martians landed in New Jersey. His adaptation went out over the Columbia Broadcasting Company's network to 151 stations nationwide. And just as H. G. Wells had depicted in his book, panic ensued, best captured in one of the first stories to report the hoax, written by George M. Mahawinney of the *Philadelphia Inquirer*. Here is his lead:

> Terror struck at the hearts of hundreds of thousands of persons in the length and breadth of the United States last night as crisp words of what they believed to be a news broadcast leaped from their radio sets, telling of catastrophe from the skies visited on this country.

The news story quoted terrified sources, including a woman in a church who screamed: "New York is destroyed; it's the end of the world. You might as well go home to die." Orson Welles proved that mass media could spark mass hysteria. But there was another important lesson about the hoax: *timing*. Remember, the year was 1938, and the day was Halloween Eve, known as "Mischief Night" in New Jersey. That may have lent the right mood. But back then Americans had been keeping a close eye on Nazi Germany, whose massive high-tech armies were ready to mobilize in Europe like Martians in Wells' book, threatening world war. Fear was rampant that year. And fear, rather than reason—upon which science and ethics are based—empowers hoaxes.

Because a diagnosis of cancer strikes fear in individuals, cancer often is a target for hoaxsters. In fact, the Food and Drug Administration has issued warnings to cancer patients, knowing that they may be "frightened by a diagnosis of cancer [and] may want to believe in the existence of 'a miracle cure.'" In an FDA article titled "Unproven Cancer Treatments: Hope or Hoax?" author Lenore Gelb notes that extravagant claims for questionable cancer treatments are often found in testimonials in the media. And the media now more than ever are perpetuating more hoaxes, primarily because hoaxsters have more ways to reach the public, using talk shows, scandal sheets, modems, faxes, 1-900 call-in numbers, and home pages. Home pages on the worldwide web often feature dozens of "testimonials" and can seem quite convincing to cancer patients fearing both diagnoses and/or mainstream treatments. The FDA cautions consumers to keep these guidelines in mind when considering questionable cancer therapies:

> **❖ Inspiration Point**
>
> **You already know the basics of gene therapy. Now you're learning fundamentals of immunotherapy. Knowing both, you should be able to discern hyped from helpful treatments, empowering yourself as a medical consumer.**

- ❖ If it sounds too good to be true, it probably is.
- ❖ Don't believe you have nothing to lose.
- ❖ Scientific medicine is accountable.

Increasingly, the American Cancer Society publishes bulletins to defuse hoaxes or explain questionable treatments, many of which are billed as "natural"—herbs or extracts—that cancer patients can administer themselves. Often the products contain names that suggest they are associated with gene therapy or mainstream cancer treatment. Beware of untested therapies that use the words "cell" or "immuno" to suggest FDA approval. Don't overlook them, either. Simply research them or contact the American Cancer Society for updated information. As always, consult a physician. To protect yourself as a health care consumer, remember the focus of this book: information eases fear and empowers you to make appropriate choices. You already know the basics of gene therapy. In this chapter you will learn the fundamentals of immunotherapy. Knowing both, you should be able to discern hyped from helpful treatments.

❧ ❧ ❧

The War of the Cells

Using the human immune system to ward off cancer is not a new idea. But recent developments concerning this therapy *are*. Nearly a century ago, researchers realized that cancer cells could elicit an immune response. This immediately sparked hope that immunotherapy might become a potent weapon in the arsenal against cancer. The hope dimmed in the 20th Century as scientists learned more about the ability of mutations to replicate and out-maneuver conventional treatments. That's why researchers usually keep their hope in check, even in the wake of advances in cancer therapy. The disease has proved a formidable opponent to generations of the best minds in medical science. Science, though, has changed in the 21st Century, partly because of such challenges as the AIDS epidemic and because of breakthroughs in both research and communication technology, allowing geneticists to peer under the cell's canopy and share discoveries worldwide. Although researchers remain cautious, respecting the common foe of cancer, they acknowledge that recent advances in gene therapy may finally realize the promise and potential of cancer immunotherapy.

As you now know, cancer cells avoid recognition and destruction by the immune system *via selected mutations.* Mutations differ from foreign invaders like bacteria because they are spawned within a person's body and thereby can elude primary natural defenses. You'll recall how the immune system "sees" foreign proteins by noticing the presence of fragments on the surface of the cells producing them. Once the immune system recognizes these "foreign" protein fragments on the cellular surface, it initiates a series of responses. The body goes to war as if a general alarm has been sounded, activating the body's defenses. The response is similar to the fictive one against the invading aliens of *The War of the Worlds.* A more apt title here might be *The War of the Cells,* with white blood cells representing humans and tumors representing aliens.

❧ ❧ ❧

The Normal Immune Response

Let's focus awhile on how your immune system should respond to a threat. Then you will be better able to understand why cancer cells can circumvent it. To begin with, one group of white blood cells—we'll call them "targeted killer cells"—is stimulated rapidly to divide upon viewing the foreign fragments on a cell's surface. The rapid division produces millions and millions of these targeted killers. In a short while they multiply into an awesome cellular army to attack and destroy the cells displaying the fragments. All well and good. Just as generals in real life have to muster or draft an army, requiring a series of steps, so too must this occur at the cellular level. For the body to muster an army of killer cells, it has to send biological signals by yet another pathway.

Enter now the "helper cells." These emanate from another group of white blood cells whose job is to send signals raising and supplying legions of targeted killer cells. Again this is similar to what occurs in the military. A real army has both front line soldiers and a supply corps upon which the soldiers depend. That is what's happening here. However, there is a hitch. These helper cells cannot be activated merely by the *presence* of foreign fragments on normal cells. Another type of white blood cell "informs" the helpers the way spies do in the intelligence branch of an army.

Spies have key functions on the real or cellular battlefield. Actual human spies go behind the front lines and collect information or capture and interrogate a few of the enemy, passing that data along to the army poised to attack. Likewise, this type of immune cell also samples the characteristics of its enemy. These clever spies are highly specialized cells that engulf other cells they believe might be foreign. In fact, they chew them up. That way they can present the protein fragments of a potential enemy on their own surface. Often they sample one of their own cells, but since these cells contain no foreign proteins, the spies who have captured their own have nothing interesting to show for their efforts. On the other hand, when these spies do gobble up a cell with foreign fragments, they present them on their own surface as if parading their capture in front of their own troops. As soon as that happens, in concert with their comrade spies, helper cells of the supply corps are activated.

Now military activity within the body picks up. The helper cells send out powerful signals calling forth more spies to further sample the supposed enemy. These signals also stimulate expansion of the targeted killer cells, which have already been activated because foreign protein fragments have been spotted on the surface of enemy cells. The combined action of the spy cells, helper cells, and killer cells—now all present in ever increasing numbers—then begin the complete destruction of the enemy cells.

That's how the immune system is supposed to work. When the enemy is cancer, however, the system cannot muster the forces needed to annihilate a malignant tumor.

❧ ❧ ❧

A Formidable Foe

Tumor cells evade the immune system's elaborate cascade of recognition and attack. Cancer cells don't present their protein fragments properly and also repel the early spy cells of the immune system. Attempts over the last decades to aid the immune system in recognizing tumor cells and mounting an attack against them have proved less than encouraging. But today's understanding of the detailed molecular mechanisms by which the immune system functions may soon change the outlook for cancer immunotherapy.

Cancer cells have many means to shield its "difference" from the immune system. At times they seem invisible. So researchers theorized moving the presentation of this "difference" away from the protective environment of the tumor itself. That's like luring an enemy division away from the camouflage of the main army, alerting the defense forces and mustering them to respond to the threat. Recently several tumor antigens—those tumor proteins that the immune system views as foreign—have been isolated from tumor cells and identified. If these antigens could be presented to the immune system at some distant site in the body, away from the shielding effects of the tumor, per-

> **❖ Inspiration Point**
>
> **Researchers have identified "super spy" cells of the body's defensive army that can trigger *all* aspects of the immune system. Excitement is generating for this new therapy which is still being tested.**

haps a normal immune response against them could be raised.

There were some early crude attempts to accomplish this objective. Researchers simply injected these proteins as classic vaccines, yielding poor results. But immunologists have learned much more about the "spies" of the immune army. The best of these spies are called dendritic (pronounced *"den-DRIT-ick"*) cells. When these highly effective spies present a foreign antigen to the immune system, the body's defenses typically swing into action. Furthermore, immunologists now know that these remarkable dendritic spy cells can activate targeted killer cells as well as helper cells. Since these "super spies" of our defensive army can trigger *all* aspects of the immune system, much attention has now been focused on them as effective agents in the fight against cancer.

In early phase clinical trials in human patients, immunologists have been able to isolate these spy cells from the blood and feed them tumor antigens. The loading of specific tumor antigens into these primed super spies allows them to present the tumor proteins as foreign proteins which activates an immune response against them. This new approach has great promise as a complex vaccination procedure to combat cancer cells. Perhaps before long antigens from a biopsy of a patient's tumor will be introduced into the dendritic spy cells of the patient. Those cells would be injected back into that patient, away from the site of the tumor, in order to raise an immune reaction against the tumor and thereby block further spread and metastasis. An even more elegant way of "loading" dendritic cells with tumor antigens to spark the body's natural immune response simply fuses together tumor cells with dendritic cells. This creates "hybrid" cells called "dendritomas," which are both dendritic and tumorous in nature. To envision how this occurs on the cellular level, imagine two soap bubbles—one a tumor cell and the other a dendritic spy cell—adhering to each other. The surfaces shimmer and quaver and then, like soap bubbles, merge into one hyrbid "dendritoma." These hybrids now are super spies that produce all the tumor proteins and contain all the tumor antigens and so can effectively show the antigens to the white blood cell army, generating killer cells. This is the hope of tumor immunologists and the reason for much of the excitement in this aspect of oncology. Yet there are several other reasons to be optimistic about the prospect of arming the immune system of a cancer patient to fire salvos at a tumor.

The Second Most Complex System

After the brain, the immune system is the most complex system of the body. Adding to this complexity are its two very different basic divisions. You may be aware that the immune system produces defensive proteins called antibodies in response to foreign molecules. That's one function. Usually only immunologists understand that your intricate immune system has a second, separate and distinct function, which attacks foreign cells. Essentially, one division of the immune system responds to and attacks foreign *molecules*, while the other does the

> ❖ **Inspiration Point**
>
> **Genetic vaccines against cancer are being considered both to block the spread of an existing primary tumor and as a protective measure against cancer in families with a high incidence of certain tumors.**

same with foreign *cells*. The first is a simple molecular recognition, but the second is more complex, requiring the call-up of the cellular defensive army. That army can only "see" foreign molecules within the context of a cell. The defensive army can see more clearly if the foreign molecule or protein is produced within a cell presenting the invader to our immune system. This characteristic of the cellular division of our defenses is logical since we evolved this aspect of our immune system to defend against clever invaders like viruses, which replicate themselves within our own cells.

This is a lot like the science fiction movie *Independence Day*—influenced by *The War of the Worlds.* (Humanity is saved again by a virus, this time a computer virus uploaded into the alien's command ship.) In *Independence Day,* invading aliens use our own satellite system to set up an attack. Invader viruses do this too, using cells rather than satellites. A defense that responds to this misuse of our cells by evil agents like viruses has protected us from such enemies for eons. The question here is, "How do you arouse the cellular aspect of our immune system to attack a cancerous growth?"

First, a few givens. The defensive army can see an invader more clearly if produced *within a cell.* Researchers know it is far better to produce tumor antigens in that manner, rather than introducing them into the body as an already made protein. Of course, this is exactly what the cancer cells are doing—reproducing themselves rapidly within cells containing mutations. Unfortunately, as we have already seen, these wily cancer cells have selected mutations that allow them to avoid immune recognition. So some *other* cell must be engineered to produce and present tumor antigens, activating the immune system against the cancer.

By now you may be able to imagine just how this can be done. Remember, gene therapy introduces selected genes into cells. The added genes produce a protein product in these cells, as you have learned in the last chapter. Gene therapy changes how we view the vaccination process. At the dawn of the genetic age, physicians vaccinating a patient will try to *stimulate* a response from the cellular division of the immune system, activating the defensive army.

❧ ❧ ❧

The New Genetic Vaccines

Already many pharmaceutical companies are testing new genetic vaccines. Instead of injecting a killed virus or some proteins from a virus into one's arm to trigger a defensive immune reaction against the virus, as is now done, this new strategy will just inject one or more of the viral genes into that same arm. Once within the cells of the patient's arm these genetic vaccines will begin producing viral proteins from within these cells, prompting the raising of super armies affording the patient much stronger protection. Genetic vaccines against cancer are being considered both to block the spread of an existing primary tumor and as a protective measure against cancer in families with a high incidence of certain tumors.

Gene therapy offers even more than the prospect of a genetic tumor vaccine. By using gene therapy it may be possible to engineer tumor cells to stop evading the immune system and to assist it in recognizing them as "foreign" and mounting an attack against themselves. This, actually, is the inciting of mutiny on the cellular battlefield, using mutations of a tumor the way real armies use counterspies. This proposed alliance between gene therapy and immune therapy has an additional appealing feature. Remember that one of the great limitations of gene therapy is its inability to introduce curative genes into a high percentage of tumor cells. Not so with the immune system. To activate it you only need to introduce genes into a small percentage of tumor cells. These few cells would then become targets for recognition, triggering the body's defenses to attack all the remaining tumor cells, even those not modified by genetic therapy. This fact makes gene therapy and immune therapy natural allies in the war against cancer.

Within the last decade, several clever strategies have been developed to utilize gene therapy to render cancer cells better targets for immunological attack. Some of these approaches have proved successful in laboratory mice and have already been moved along into human clinical trials. Each approach attempts to utilize gene therapy to activate a particular aspect of the natural immune response.

Some tumor immunologists argue that in many tumors cancer cells present foreign fragments on their surface. The problem (they believe) is that cancer cells activate immune cells with these fragments only *weakly*. So only a relative few killer cells are mustered and represent no match on the cellular battlefield. These immunologists also contend that such tumors are not destroyed by these killers because no helper cells are activated to provide the necessary signals to raise a formidable defensive army. But what if tumor cells, somehow, could be engineered to produce the signals along with a strong immune response?

These researchers set out to accomplish just that. Their objective was the signal that activates the killer cells. The technical name of that signal is Interleukin 2 (pronounced *"IN-ter-LUKE-in"*) or IL-2. First in laboratory experiments with mice and then in a series of human clinical trials, the IL-2 gene was introduced by gene therapy into tumor cells. Researchers noted a significant immune response against all the cells of many of these tumors. Moreover, the introduction of the IL-2 gene into only a few tumor cells was sufficient to stimulate the immune response against the whole tumor. This response was shown to be the result of a much more effective stimulation, triggering massive expansion of killer cells.

Another therapy is based on a different assumption. That is, the principal means by which tumor cells avoid immune surveillance is by keeping the "spy" cells from their midst. In other words, the tumor renders the entire defensive army useless because that army lacks spies. And as in real life, an army without information is also a defeated one on the battlefield. In this new approach, researchers are trying to use gene therapy to *recruit* spy cells into the tumor. This is done through the introduction of the gene for GMCSF, otherwise known as granulocyte macrophage colony stimulating factor (pronounced *"GRAN-yoo-LOW-site MACK-re-fage"*). The added gene produces this signaling protein, which attracts and recruits spy cells into cancer cells. In studies using this method, a large influx of spy cells was attracted to the tumors and a substantial immune response to the tumors was generated by the patient's immune system.

Both of these approaches, employing IL-2 and GMCSF, lead to all-out warfare between the immune system's defensive army and tumor cells. While the results are very encouraging, neither method can mount a strong enough immune response to counter the expanding mass of established tumors. But as in every war, there is usually another battle on the horizon. And again there is cause for tempered hope.

❧ ❧ ❧

The Special Case of Leukemia

Because blood is a fluid tissue, cancers like leukemia—associated with the cellular tributaries of the blood system—have different features from the solid tumors of other tissues. In some sense, leukemia represents "The War of the *Naval* Cells." This makes discussion of leukemia a special case in which immunotherapy may play a key role in the future.

Because leukemia often strikes children, it is truly an affront to our sense of fairness. Offsetting this, however, is the fact that leukemia is one of the most treatable cancers using available present-day chemotherapy. This is an important point, because as you already know, standard chemotherapy is not always effective with other cancers spawning solid tumors.

> **❖ Inspiration Point**
>
> **Many of the advanced therapies offer hope of gentler treatments for leukemia patients. The most promising of the new treatments for leukemia involve immunotherapy.**

To understand this difference, you might remember the discussion in the second chapter concerning how normal healthy tissues maintain a constant cellular population. You were asked to envision orchards of beautiful trees—some that drop seed-cones, others that drop seed-propellers, and still others that drop seeds from flowers on limbs. Some of these trees like corkscrew willows don't even need to drop cones, propellers, or seeds but simply sprout offspring from shoots. Every so often healthy tissues sprout new "seedling" cells, which then divide a prerequisite number of times before succumbing to programmed cell death . . . only to be replaced by new "seedling" cells in a carefully choreographed eternal harvest. Biologists understand this complex process well, especially as it applies to the blood system. So, they were able to fathom the complexities of leukemia and recommend highly effective treatments.

Remember, the warfare here plays out as if on water. Cellular scientists have charted the detailed channels by which a small number of "seeding" cells, called stem cells, expand and specialize into the many different cell types of our blood system. To attack the cancer, physicians essentially destroy the waterways of the entire blood system, including armadas of cancer cells. They use radiation or chemotherapy to do this and then replenish the "seas" of the blood system, transplanting new healthy stem cells from a donor into the patient's blood system.

The replacement cells are taken from the donor's bone marrow. So this procedure became known as "bone marrow transplantation." When a matched donor can be found with cells the patient will not reject, the procedure successfully treats leukemia. But finding a matched donor is rare, and the procedure places the patient in significant risk. Until the transplant takes hold, patients must survive for a period without a functioning blood or immune system.

Because of these drawbacks, oncologists specializing in treating leukemia began focusing on the use of the patient's own stem cells. This only seemed natural. After all, true stem cells rarely divide and also have the capacity to completely rebuild a patient's blood system. So they are not a part of the cancer process and, better yet, are also almost completely resistant to the ravages of chemotherapeutic drugs that target healthy and cancerous cells, destroying the entire cellular "seas" of the blood system. Oncologists thought, why not destroy the blood system using very high doses of radiation or chemotherapy, killing the cancer armadas, and then use the patient's own stem cells like tributaries to replenish those "seas" with pristine waters?

In principal, such a strategy should work. But there was a big hurdle. Even with support from transfusions, patients without a functional blood system receiving such treatment would not survive long enough to replenish their systems. However, the good news is that the procedure was modified somewhat and now is highly effective. Two advancements made these modified "self-transplants" possible. First, researchers were able to identify and isolate stem cells at "middle age," when they are most useful for transplantation purposes. This occurs when they are at a stage between true blood stem cells and their mature descendants. Researchers also discovered natural molecules, called cytokines (pronounced *"SITE-oh-kines"*), which speed the maturation of stem cells and these intermediate cells, again advancing them to their most useful stage, when they can rebuild the blood system most effectively.

These advances have occurred because of a cellular vision. The emerging biotechnology industry is almost solely responsible for such progress, now producing cytokine drugs. The industry also has invented a storage system, using specialized equipment to isolate the intermediate blood cell "precursors" (rebuilders) from a patient's blood. This way the valuable cells that can replenish the seas of the blood system may be stored during the intense radiation or chemotherapy used to destroy the patient's blood and tumor cells. After such treatment, those intermediate, cancer-free blood cells are returned to the patient who receives the powerful cytokines. These drugs speed the rebuilding of the blood system because the intermediate cells act as a stop gap while true stem cells re-establish the natural cycles of tissue restoration.

Chemotherapy or radiation therapy is more effective in treating leukemia than other cancers because leukemia afflicts the blood. Higher doses of traditional therapies can be used without endangering the patient because the damaged tissue (blood) can be restored naturally. Despite advances, chemotherapy and radiation treatment are harsh treatments, especially when administered to children. Many of the advanced therapies discussed here and in the next chapter offer hope of gentler treatments for leukemia patients.

The most promising of the new treatments for leukemia involves immunotherapy. Because leukemia is a special case, such treatments are approached differently from immunotherapy for other tumors. In essence, leukemia is a disease of the cells of the immune system. Since the patient's immune function is often impaired or skewed by this disease, generating an immune response *to* the disease may require circumventing the natural immune system. Therefore, an immune response to leukemia may have to be generated in the laboratory and transferred to the patient. Early indication that such a complex immune therapy might work for leukemia patients comes from bone marrow transplantation therapy.

When a leukemia patient receives a bone marrow transplant from a donor, the match is almost never perfect and some rejection occurs. Most people think that the patient rejects the transplanted immune system. It's the other way around. The newly transplanted immune system rejects the patient's tissues. At first physicians tried to block or mask that rejection. Then they noted that the new immune system was responding not only against the patient's tissues, but also against the patient's leukemia cells. This reaction, called a "graft vs. leukemia response" to the transplant, was shown to be a powerful ally in combating leukemia. This "graft vs. leukemia" response is the result of the immune killer cells of the patient's new defensive navies attacking the cancer. Unfortunately, the patient's own immune system does not seem to mount any significant similar response against the tumor. But scientists and physicians are now attempting to stimulate some of the crews of the patient's defensive navy away from the cancer. By creating and expanding a navy of killer white blood cells targeted against the leukemia and re-introducing this combat force back into the patient, researchers hope to generate a strong "self graft vs. leukemia" response. This approach is quite promising and soon may provide a "gentler" approach to the treatment of this disease.

In sum, the promise of immunotherapy has been enhanced by the emergence of gene therapy as an effective new tool in the hands of the physician. *Gene therapy, immunotherapy and their combination will surely change the face of cancer therapy in the 21st Century.* This *face* will not be a hyped media one, but a human one in a hospital or cancer clinic. The patient will have more trust in scientifically sound therapies or combinations of therapies. This trust between the cancer team and the patient will be based on another combination: accountable science and clear conscience.

❧ ❧ ❧

Compassion

The War of the Worlds by H. G. Wells was influenced not by fiction but by philosophy. Namely *Culture and Anarchy* by English poet and scholar Matthew Arnold, who often wrote about the relationship between literature and science. Arnold believed people, regardless of class background or origin, possessed two selves: "ordinary" and "best." The ordinary self was interested in gratification. Quick fixes. It feared easily and got angry out of ignorance. We all know about this side of our nature. The best self, however, was interested in higher truths and humane spirit. The best self trusted intellect and had compassion for others. It awakened the part of ourselves about which we are most proud—those times when we have overcome the ordinariness of fear, anger, false hope, or blind faith.

Those feelings often are involved in health-care issues. We need our best self especially when the stakes are high, as they often are when dealing with cancer. *Compassion* is an ethical concept that awakens the best self. A compassionate person wants to do what many doctors, researchers, and ethicists want to do—ease the suffering, difficulties, or burdens of others. A compassionate person also forgives others easily because he or she not only knows facts but also balances them with feelings. For instance, a compassionate person feeling disabused in a hospital bed might acknowledge that the intern on call has been on rounds for thirty hours and therefore might be abrupt. Of course, that knowledge won't stop this patient from asking that harried intern a question about treatment or medicine. The patient just won't respond angrily if the information is presented in less than a cordial manner. As you can see, a person guided by the best self weighs situations and circumstances carefully because he or she not only has respect for others, but also for him- or herself.

Compassion shows a high level of awareness. Fear clouds awareness. So does anger. False hope and blind faith—in a questionable or untested treatment, for instance—erodes trust when results are not to our immediate liking. All this affects our attitude.

❦ ❦ ❦

Envisioning Exercise

Exploring Your Best Self

Objective: Restore *inner* calm to face *outer* challenges.

To come in touch with your *best self,* remember times when others expected you to act in an ordinary way . . . and you didn't. Someone might have confronted you. Instead of becoming angry or growing fearful in this situation, you responded philosophically or compassionately or acknowledged the higher truths of a situation. Begin with your earliest memories, perhaps in elementary school, and continue until the current day. Again, use a journal or tape recorder or simply contemplate or share your memories with loved ones. Try to recall at least a dozen incidents.

Ask yourself:

- ❖ When I reacted to a challenging situation with my *best self,* how did the other person respond?
- ❖ What facts did I know about the situation that played a role in my philosophical or compassionate response?
- ❖ How did I feel about myself after responding so reasonably to the challenge or situation?
- ❖ How can I revive those positive feelings now?

Of course, there will be times when you acted ordinarily and out of anger or fear when facing a challenge or confrontation. The *best self* wants to remember those moments, too, because you can relive and correct them with your imagination.

Ask yourself:

- When I reacted to a challenging situation with my *ordinary self,* how did the other person respond?
- What facts did I *lack* about the situation and what role did that play in my angry or fearful response?
- How did I feel about myself after responding so angrily or fearfully to the challenge or situation?
- How would I change those situations and feelings if I could relive them today, using my best self?

You can also base a poem, story, painting, sculpture, or some other creative work on answers to questions about the ordinary self above. That's part of the process of self forgiveness and restored trust in the higher nature of your conscience. The goal is to restore inner calm to face outer challenges, knowing that you already have the resources to do so.

Chapter Nine

❦ ❦ ❦

The New Cancer Chemotherapy

Now we have found new cracks, new weaknesses in the sheer and bleak stone face of cancer. We have wedged these cracks open. Now we are trying to widen them. And the hope, of course, is to burst through them.

—Steven A. Rosenberg, M.D., Ph.D. (1940-)

Before discussing powerful new drugs in the war against cancer, you should know how ethicists regard the concept of "power." They don't think of it in political terms, even though you hear the words "political power" every night on the news. Neither do they think of it in sporting terms, the "power" of an athlete to dominate others or the "power play" of a hockey team with one or more extra players than opponents on the ice. Ethicists tend to view "power" the way that scientists do, as a *force*. Think of "electrical power" supplied by your local "power plant." When you plug in the cord of your computer, you're not tapping into the electrical outlet but the energy that flows through it. Likewise power is not a value, according to ethicists, *but the force with which we put forth our values*. Too little, and others take advantage of us. Too much, and we oppress others. The goal of ethics is to exert precisely enough power to resolve a problem without creating greater problems. Keep this concept in mind as you contemplate the difference between traditional and new chemotherapies.

Traditional chemotherapy relies on brute force. It exerts so much power to kill tumor cells that it ends up killing healthy cells. It oppresses the body. It oppresses the patient, causing sickening side effects. The intent is to wage all-out biological warfare, poisoning the body's cells in the hope that doing so will destroy tumor cells at a somewhat faster rate than other cells.

This, alas, is a somewhat barbaric way to annihilate cancer. True, cancer involves the "The War of the Cells," but current chemotherapy is much like primitive Viking warfare in which massive warriors marched upon their enemies swinging great combat hammers. No doubt about destruction, here. Nor sheer muscle power. No hint in history that Vikings, magnificent though they were, did not oppress their enemies. Imagine a sea of six-foot-plus horned and helmeted men wielding these weapons in an enemy town and striking down people, animals, and even houses. Vikings may have won the war, but little of value remained intact afterward. Often this is the case following present-day chemotherapy when the patient is almost as debilitated by the treatment as he or she has been by the disease.

> **❖ Inspiration Point**
>
> **One of the most important goals of cancer research is to turn the tables on tumor cells, replacing the crude war hammers of current chemotherapy with new therapies and approaches that feature minimal side-effects.**

You remember those laser weapons foreseen decades before their invention in H. G. Wells' *The War of the Worlds*? When the aliens used them in the novel, the futuristic beams struck terror in everyone's heart and human armies collapsed in fear. One of the most important goals of cancer research is to turn the tables on tumor cells, replacing the crude war hammers of current chemotherapy with the metaphoric piercing light of laser weapons. That's a rather ethical approach, too, exerting power with pinpoint precision. In solving a medical problem without creating greater ones, physicians will kill cancer with minimal side effects or even render tumor cells normal again without harming any neighboring healthy cells. This lofty goal will be achieved not via brute force but via logic, based on data recently assembled about the molecular mechanisms that initiate cancer and allow it to progress.

All this has occurred because of a significant change in attitude. For instance, drugs used in medicine today usually rely on small molecules designed to either treat the cause or the symptoms of a disease or disorder. This includes such common disorders as high blood pressure, high cholesterol levels, and chronic head pain. Cancer, likewise, is now treated with small-molecule drugs that have distinct targets.

Researchers who helped design these new drugs had enhanced vision. First, they took into account each molecular event that must occur for a cancer cell to keep duplicating so quickly. After all, the tumor's ability to replicate wildly is what makes cancer so potentially lethal. In analyzing this process, researchers found small cracks in the armor of cancer cells. Second, researchers knew that cancer has to avoid destruction by the body's many natural safeguards. So in part they based the design of their drugs on this, too. By understanding how cancer replicates and avoids destruction, these researchers were able to engineer chemical agents to act on tumors with laser-like accuracy.

By now you, too, should be able to envision a few ready targets of new anti-tumor drugs. Hundreds of such drugs are being developed in both the pharmaceutical and emerging biotechnology industries. You'll learn the logic behind a few such drugs here, to give you a sense of the excitement and hope emanating out of such development.

❧ ❧ ❧

Molecular Decoys

Colorectal cancer is widespread and prevalent throughout the population. Because the detailed molecular steps by which this cancer forms are now reasonably well known, colorectal cancer has become an early target for the new class of anti-tumor drugs.

> **❖ Inspiration Point**
>
> **In the not-too-distant future, patients exhibiting early signs of colorectal cancer may receive medication to stop polyp formation and block progression to cancer. The treatment would be very much like the treatment for high blood pressure, with minimal fear attached to the diagnosis.**

Let's review a few basics about colorectal cancer, described in detail in Chapter Four. You may recall that a mutation in the APC gene of the cells lining the intestinal tract results in the over-expression of the protein COX-2. The excess COX-2 protein then interferes with the programmed cell-death safeguard of these naturally rapidly dividing cells. This often leads to the formation of polyps, an early condition that can easily lead to cancer. Several pharmaceutical companies have targeted this first step in the twisted pathway toward colorectal cancer. They are developing drugs to block the action of excess COX-2. When they do, affected polyps should return to normal tissue.

The logic is pristine. COX-2 is an enzyme that converts a simple metabolite (pronounced *"met-AB-oh-lite"*), or kind of cellular food, into a more complex byproduct. It's a lot like your body turning carbohydrates into energy. So COX-2 is drawn to that simple metabolite. By designing a small molecule that looks to COX-2 like this metabolite, drug companies hope to fool the enzyme into selectively reacting with this decoy. Of course, this decoy molecule will have other characteristics that can inhibit the action of COX-2 once it has been bound to it.

In other words, researchers working with these drug companies hope to do some "molecular fishing." Think about it. When anglers go fishing they also use decoys. A fly fisherman carefully ties a decoy-insect made of colored thread onto a sharp hook. He or she then skillfully skips the decoy over the top of the water where fish may be. If the angler is lucky, the fish bites at the decoy fly but closes his mouth onto the hook. This is exactly what the pharmaceutical scientist is trying to do, using a decoy for the metabolite that COX-2 usually "bites." If these scientists are lucky in the lab, they just may "catch" a life-saving anti-cancer drug. Already several candidates for a perfect decoy for COX-2 have been identified. An approved drug for the treatment of osteoarthritis, rofecoxib (Vioxx), is one of these candidates and has recently been shown to stop polyp formation in mice.

People at high risk because of a family history of colorectal cancer or anyone over 50 years of age should have routine rectal examinations for the appearance of polyps in their colon. A drug such as Vioxx could be used routinely to treat colorectal cancer. Here's how it would work. A physician observes the appearance of polyps and the very beginnings of the process towards colorectal cancer. Even though the patient would still be far from cancer, or any real and present danger, an oncologist would be able to prescribe Vioxx or another such COX-2 inhibitor to stop polyp formation and block its progression on to cancer. In this case, treatment for such an early diagnosis of this pre-cancerous condition would be very much like the treatment for high blood pressure. The patient would simply take a pill each day for a while or for the remainder of his or her life.

Imagine the progress, from early diagnosis to application of this new chemotherapy. This new drug could reduce a former life-threatening situation to a simple and common treatment—with *no fear* associated with that treatment. It would be tantamount to pointing laser guns at seas of invading Vikings, exploding their war hammers into splinters. And because such drugs would be prescribed to prevent cancer, drugs like COX-2 inhibitors are known as "chemopreventative" rather than chemotherapeutic drugs. And there is more good news to come. The COX-2 inhibitors are just the tip of a sparkling genetic iceberg in the new age of chemotherapy.

Case in point: Chronic myelogenous leukemia (CML) strikes 4,300 people every year in the United States. This diagnosis, like any other cancer diagnosis, typically brings instant dread as the patient is told that his or her body has lost control of the proliferation of white blood cells, allowing the cancer to take over. But, as you have come to anticipate, there is hope—so much hope, in fact, that researchers believe this type of leukemia may be successfully treated with new therapies.

CML occurs as a result of a "translocation mutation." That term, as you may recall, describes what happens when a piece of one chromosome breaks off and attaches to another chromosome, making an odd and dangerous genetic combination—like a metaphoric Ferrari pulling a manure spreader. The translocation that causes this type of leukemia fuses, quite literally, a broken chromosome called "Bcr" (the Ferrari) with another called Abl (the manure spreader). That generates the mutant "Bcr-Abl kinase."

Bcr-Abl kinase is a runaway enzyme. It is as if the Ferrari with the manure spreader, a potent if bizarre mechanical symbol, accelerates on super-high octane fuel, causing the Ferrari-spreader to run wild. This mutant enzyme keeps signaling cells to keep dividing seemingly without end, causing a heretofore-deadly cancer. In other words, the Bcr-Abl gene is always "on." The Ferrari never stops running. So the proliferation of dysfunctional white blood cells containing this mutation creates the patient's leukemia.

Because of their knowledge of the molecular events that lead to this cancer, scientists have used the "molecular fishing" approach described earlier. They have designed a drug—or a decoy, as in fishing—to inhibit the action of the mutant Bcr-Abl kinase. The result? Dramatic reductions of white blood cell proliferation and, in some cases, complete elimination of all the cells in a patient's body with the chromosome abnormality.

For the first time in the memory of cancer researchers, the term "cure" has tentatively begun to be heard associated with this new chemotherapeutic treatment.

Before this treatment, patients with chronic myelogenous leukemia usually received high doses of chemotherapy often combined with a bone marrow transplant. Even so, these individuals usually lived only 5 to 7 years after diagnosis. Not only does this new therapy lack the toxic and debilitating side effects of the prior treatment, but it also is reversing and in some cases curing this disease.

Other Chemopreventative Drugs

Consider another familiar target of chemopreventative drugs. In the second chapter of this book you learned how the cell cycle is regulated. You may recall that many of the important regulatory proteins affect the cell cycle's action proteins—the cellular machinery that splits magic logs not into two halves but into two new logs. You remember this happens when certain "mechanic" proteins spray phosphates on them. We called those mechanics "cyclin dependent kinases," or CDKs, but we never discussed where they got the phosphates from in the first place. Well, they get them from another simple metabolite called ATP. Once they fill their canisters, they can spray their chemical on the action proteins, starting up the cellular machinery to cut those "logs" and make duplicate cells. You'll also remember that cell replication can go out of control when cancer occurs, as if one of those foreman gatekeepers collapses at the cellular assembly line, allowing the factory to fill up to the ceiling and beyond with magic logs because no one can find the "off" switch. In other words, those spray-can mechanics keep filling up on that metabolite ATP. What if a drug could be designed so that the mechanics filled up their canisters with a decoy equivalent?

Of course, scientists searching for that decoy know that there are many regulatory proteins of the body. Each is slightly different. Worse, the portion of these proteins that binds the ATP metabolite—essentially allowing the "mechanic" to fill up the spray canister—is also only subtly dissimilar. But this is a crack in the stone face of cancer, and researchers want to exploit it. To do it, pharmaceutical scientists are designing "ATP decoys" that target specific regulators of the cell cycle that activate replication in cancer cells. At one time, this challenge seemed overwhelming because of the subtle differences between all these similar phosphate-transferring proteins. But research scientists have made remarkable progress in accomplishing this feat. The new drugs that they have discovered can block the activation of cell cycling in specific tumor cells in laboratory mice—without inhibiting normal cellular activity or resulting in any side effects. Everyone in oncology is excited about upcoming clinical trials. If successful, these regulatory drugs can be used to treat several types of cancers.

Researchers have embarked on more "fishing" expeditions, using molecular decoys. Remember the RAS protein, that carrier pigeon from Chapter Four, dropping messages to produce an overabundance of 'drivers" that stimulated the cell cycle? You'll recall that the RAS protein was over-expressed as a result of a mutation in its gene, making it instrumental in the second step of colorectal cancer from polyps to early stage adenomas. What we didn't cover was the over-expression of the RAS protein being associated not only with colorectal cancer but also with many other cancers. But RAS is different from other activators of the cell cycle. First and foremost, it does not act directly at the site of the cell-cycle machinery. After RAS is produced within the cell it is transported to the cell's outer surface. That's a distinguishing feature, and all such features are potential targets of the new chemotherapy, because scientists can disrupt the cellular process by honing in or decoying that special feature. When RAS is transported to the cell's outer surface, it then receives signals from factors in the blood stream and relays them to the cell-cycle machinery, thereby strongly stimulating it. But here's the hitch, indicating another crack in the stone face of cancer; for RAS to be transported to the cell surface and to remain there, a "fatty tail" must be attached to this protein molecule. All this takes place in the cell's outer membrane, an "outer skin" enclosing and containing the somewhat spherically shaped watery sea of proteins and other molecules that make up a cell. This membrane is a structure not unlike the surface of the soap bubbles a child might blow from a loop dipped into a soap solution. This "soapy" surface of our cells soaks up fatty materials just like dish soap soaks up the fats on dirty dishes. This is why the addition of a fatty tail to RAS sends it directly to the outer membrane of the cell and holds it there. Pharmaceutical scientists have built decoys that inhibit the transfer of the fatty tail to RAS, keeping it from moving to the cell surface and thereby completely blocking its action. These drugs have real promise for all those cancers in which RAS is one of the principal simulators of wild cellular proliferation. Because each of these molecular decoys is a small molecule, these drugs can be taken orally and can reach each and every cancer cell. But because they are so targeted for a specific molecular event within the cancer cell they have little or no side effects on the patient's normal cells. Again the result is a new chemotherapy that features laser-like precision weapons. Only tumor cells, not people, will fear such a treatment.

❧ ❧ ❧

Blockading the Tumor

Tumor cells are insidious. Not only do they master stealth and evade the body's natural defenses, they rely on assistance from non-tumor cells that act like traitors, betraying the body. No tumor larger than a few cubic millimeters can survive on its own. It needs an extensive vascular system that supplies blood so the cancerous mass can grow. The tumor's vascular tentacles are not made up of rapidly proliferating cancer cells that have the ability to mutate swiftly around natural or man-made defenses. This is a *new* blood vessel formation, feeding the cancer and subverting normal cells of the normal life process. To set up such a traitorous formation, new vessels emerge from pre-existing blood vessels. This is called angiogenesis (pronounced *"AN-jee-oh-JEN-ah-sis"*). Normally angiogenesis is only associated with the body's natural wound-healing process. In a real sense, the tumor recruits it to its cause.

In healthy adults, angiogenesis occurs slowly and infrequently. The turnover of the cells in blood vessels happens on the order of *years*. This is yet another crack in the stone face of cancer. Here's why: temporary elimination of angiogenesis would clearly inhibit the growth of any solid tumor mass by robbing it of its nutrients; moreover, such a strategy would not likely result in any serious effects on the normal life process. For this reason an increasing number of cancer scientists now believe that tumor angiogenesis offers an opportunity to target a cellular opponent—those traitor cells—which cannot escape via mutation and stealth associated with

❖ Inspiration Point

No tumor larger than a few cubic millimeters can survive on its own. Temporary elimination of blood vessel formation would clearly inhibit the growth of any solid tumor mass by robbing it of its nutrients; moreover, such a strategy would not likely result in any serious effects for the patient.

rapidly dividing tumor cells. If the new blood vessel formation upon which tumors depend could be inhibited, the tumor should die away without the side effects of traditional chemotherapy. In sum, such an approach would "blockade" the tumor the way defensive navies blockade an enemy nation, depriving it of its needs. This is the logic behind one of the most exciting and novel contemporary approaches to the treatment of cancer. Currently specialized molecular drugs are being developed that can block the formation of blood vessels that feed tumors.

There's more good news on the immediate horizon. Advances in tumor biology, which led to this innovative approach to treat cancer, have taken place concurrently with dramatic progress in our understanding of the cellular process by which blood vessels are formed. All this now offers several options to inhibit or halt tumor angiogenesis. To appreciate the logic of these approaches, however, you need to know more about the cellular land- and seascape associated with blood-vessel formation.

As you know by now, the life process is awesome. One of its most wondrous aspects concerns how individual cells self-assemble into complex three-dimensional structures. These structures form the functional tissues of our bodies. They literally make you what you are, a 3-dimensional being of consciousness with intricate organs and systems networking with other organs and systems. All this begins at the cellular level, and blood-vessel formation is a classic example of this striking cellular *self*-organization.

Normally such cellular assembly occurs during early embryonic development. Detailed studies of the molecular and cellular mechanisms that trigger self-assembly are now possible and serve as the basis for the modern science of developmental biology. Studies of the early processes of cellular organization in the formation of animal and human tissues have led to an understanding of how blood vessel formation takes place. This knowledge may well lead to a highly effective treatment for cancer.

There is, however, an ethical consideration concerning use of embryonic tissue for research purposes. As all ethicists know, controversial issues should not be oversimplified. There are always competing interests. The more controversial the issue, the higher the stakes. Thus, those who question the appropriateness of studying early human development and uses of embryonic tissue for this purpose should weigh their concerns against the medical value of such studies that may lead, finally, to the conquest of cancer.

The biological issues here are also complex. As mentioned earlier, the formation of blood vessels through angiogenesis is a rare occurrence in a healthy adult. But during some of the earliest phases of embryo formation the rapid and prolific formation of blood vessels is important and necessary for the survival of the growing embryo. This early production of blood vessels is slightly different from adult angiogenesis and is known as vasculogenesis (pronounced *"VAS-cue-loh-JEN-ah-sis"*). Nonetheless, many features of these processes are identical.

Much that is known today about angiogenesis has been learned from the study of embryonic vasculogenesis. At the dawning of life within the womb, large numbers of cells, which appear in every way just like any other embryonic cells, suddenly begin to assemble, as if by magic, into a network of inner-connecting tubes that carry the newly formed blood cells throughout the body of the developing fetus. Scientists studying this remarkable process now have more insight into the molecular events that drive this miraculous cellular assembly.

Beneath the cellular landscape of vasculogenesis and angiogenesis lies the complex molecular machinery of the endothelial (pronounced *"END-oh-THEEL-ee-all"*) cells. These cells form our blood vessels. Developmental biologists studying these processes have now begun to unravel the details of this molecular machinery that sparks the assembly of our veins, arteries, and tiny capillaries. The embryonic endothelial cells remain dissociated in random pools of cellular units until their genome begins to express the protein integrin. As integrin begins to be produced within these cells it migrates to the cell surface where it affixes itself to the outer surface of the endothelial cells. Once the endothelial cells are decorated with integrin on their outer surface this important protein begins to direct their self-assembly into tubes. Integrin binds strongly to a class of proteins known as extra-cellular matrix proteins. This is the "stuff" that coats the outer surface of many cells, including those of our blood vessels. These matrix proteins include the protein "collagen," promoted as a natural agent of youthful skin, as well as many other less well-known proteins. Some of these proteins include fibronectin, so named because it is a fibrous protein connecting cells together, and laminin, so named because it "laminates" cells together. These long fibrous extra-cellular proteins bind to the newly expressed integrin molecules on the surface of the embryonic endothelial cells. That causes them to weave together into tubular sheets.

Essentially the same molecular process also drives angiogenesis in healthy adults. Knowledge of this process allowed cancer scientists to devise a strategy to block tumor angiogenesis. Cancer scientists argued that the extra cellular matrix proteins—fibronectin and laminin—probably were molecular bridges between the cells that make up the tumor's blood vessels. It was only logical. After all, these matrix proteins bound to the important organizing integrin proteins on the outside of the endothelial cells involved in tumor angiogenesis. A bridge existed somewhere, these scientists knew, and those matrix proteins were a good bet. In cellular warfare, as in human warfare, bridges are key targets. So these scientists then devised a clever way to keep these "bridges" from forming between the endothelial cells, effectively blocking the formation of tumor blood vessels.

Researchers envisioned a cellular blockade to starve the tumor into submission. They assumed that one end of a collagen molecule bound to the integrin on one endothelial cell. That's one part of the "bridge." But the bridge was not yet complete. Remember, this is an intricately woven pattern of bridgework much like the criss-crossing "canals" on Mars. Thus, the bridging molecule was also bound to the integrin on an adjacent endothelial cell, connecting them into a *continuous tublar structure.*

How might scientists block this essential cellular cross-linking? One group introduced a fragment of the collagen protein that only contained the end that could bind to one cell, but lacked the other end to complete the cross-link. In this way, they theorized, all the integrins on the endothelial cells would be bound by a collagen fragment, but none would be crossed-linked. This is like the closing of key locks in a complex canal system. Boats just can't get through. While this idea seems almost too simple to work, remarkably, these collagen fragments very effectively blocked tumor angiogenesis in laboratory animals.

These collagen fragments are called endostatin (pronounced *"END-oh-STAT-in"*). They are so named because they stop endothelial cells from forming vascular structures. These fragments will soon be used in clinical trials to block the growth and spread of cancers in human patients. Cancer researchers are especially hopeful about this therapy since it targets normal endothelial cells that are less likely than wily cancer cells to break through this molecular blockade.

❧ ❧ ❧

Hope for Breast and Prostate Cancers

As stressed throughout this book, cancer is not a single disease but a class of diseases. This makes each cancer different. Some cancers are very aggressive. So cells of these tumors must either be destroyed or have their defect corrected as soon as possible. Other cancers are much slower in their progression. These tumors often can be kept in check, simply by reducing factors that stimulate the cell cycle.

Two cancers, in particular, have certain marked similarities, although they usually affect opposite sexes: prostate cancer and breast cancer. The cells from which each of these tumors are derived come from 'sexual" tissues. In other words, the growth of each of these tumors is strongly stimulated by sex hormones. In the case of breast cancer, the tumor cell cycle is often stimulated by estrogen. In prostate cancer it is testosterone, the male sex hormone. If some patients with slow-progressing breast or prostate cancer are placed upon a regimen of sex hormone inhibitors, their tumors can often be controlled.

As you have come to anticipate by now, there is always some challenge that researchers have to take into consideration for drug therapy to be effective. In the case of breast and prostate cancer, it is often the patient's attitude. You can anticipate the problem on a personal level. Not only is the patient deeply depressed upon learning about a cancer diagnosis but also often despondent to know that he or she may also lose many aspects of sexuality. Sometimes the specter of this double loss causes a patient to refuse a treatment that might otherwise save his or her life.

Many researchers are sensitive to this situation and have made it the focus of yet another drug-development strategy. The proteins that bind to sex hormones in tumor cells are often subtly different from those proteins that bind to the same hormones, stimulating "manly" or "womanly" characteristics. These include breast development in women and muscle formation in men and libido in both. Of course, these directly affect the expressions of our sexuality. Several pharmaceutical companies are pursuing "decoy" drugs that can inhibit sex hormone activation of tumors of sexual tissue, but not block normal sexual expression. Currently being tested are several selective estrogen inhibitors for the treatment of breast cancer. These drugs do not inhibit femininity. Not far behind in the laboratory are similar drugs for prostate cancer.

❧ ❧ ❧

Engineering the End of Cancer

It is only fitting that *Living Without Fear* conclude with a vision of victory—your own, perhaps, but also one over cancer. Researchers are working tirelessly toward that goal, exploring and testing concepts that emanate out of human consciousness—the crowning jewel of our species. We believe that the war against cancer is likely to be won not by labs equipped with futuristic technology but by researchers equipped with visionary approaches.

So far we have covered approaches involving "molecular fishing" with decoy molecules. There are other approaches, of course, being developed in the testing and production of the next generation of chemotherapeutic drugs. Perhaps one of the most exciting areas of new anti-tumor drug development involves an entirely new class of pharmaceuticals. Again you're going to appreciate the scientific mind at work, using the laser beams of logic instead of the Viking war hammers of yore to treat and prevent cancer.

> **❖ Inspiration Point**
>
> **DNA is one of life's mysterious most intricate creations. Nonetheless, the time is approaching when researchers will design selective drugs like the molecular decoys to act directly upon this molecule of life.**

As you well know by now, cancer is a disease of the DNA molecule and as such is very different from other diseases. So if drugs that truly inhibit cancer are to be developed, then it is likely that some of these must act directly upon the DNA molecule. Of course, most existing traditional chemotherapeutic drugs do act upon DNA but rather sledgehammer it to trigger a cell-death program that is ineffective when the gatekeeper suppressor, known as "p53," has a mutation. And DNA is one of life's mysterious most intricate creations. Nonetheless, the time is approaching when researchers will design selective drugs like the molecular decoys to act directly upon the molecule of life.

Already, the first steps toward such drugs have been taken. But how can drugs be selective for a certain gene involved in cancer and not affect other genes or other parts of the vast genetic molecular garden of DNA? To address this, you have to ask, "What is special about the molecule of life?" And that answer is easy: its shape. Unlike proteins that each have a different shape and a slightly different "pocket"—a kind of stomach where they consume the cellular food of metabolites—the shape and structure of DNA is simple and unchanged throughout its length. DNA is DNA is DNA. This incredibly long molecule viewed under the electron microscope looks like an unending railroad track going off into eternity with one segment identical to any other. Another distinct characteristic of DNA is its language. You'll remember that the basis of difference between genes is the *sequence* of the four different units used to encode genetic information. Again, logic comes into play. The only possible means by which a molecule could be designed to selectively interact and inhibit one gene—while not affecting others—is for that molecule to be able to *recognize* the unique sequence of units within a gene. Could such molecules be designed? Logic says "yes."

Here's why. We know that such molecular recognition is possible since signaling proteins act by binding to the regulatory regions of genes. When they do, they recognize their sequence. This way, they can regulate and orchestrate gene expression. The real issue is not whether the approach would work against cancer, but whether geneticists can engineer such complex molecules.

The first hurdle is size. Drugs the size of the molecular decoys already discussed are far too small to be able to "see" enough of the sequence of a gene to recognize and bind to it. So if molecules that can recognize selected genes can be designed they will have to be larger molecules. In fact, it is likely that they will have to be *polymeric* molecules—in other words, chemically similar to DNA—like the genetic regulatory proteins that recognize gene sequences. Several groups of chemists have begun to synthesize manmade polymers that have some ability to recognize DNA sequence. These molecules are most likely the forerunners of the ultimate anti-tumor drugs. If such molecules can be designed to recognize the regulatory regions of genes—for instance, the cyclin dependent kinase "driver" gene of cellular proliferation—many new vistas will open to effective cancer drug therapy. The current thinking goes like this: perhaps such molecules could bind selectively to mutated regulatory sequences in the driver gene. In other words, it will hone in laser-like to the damaged cellular roadway of DNA. Maybe the manmade molecules will block the activation of oncogenes by targeting and suppressing the genes of regulatory proteins that stimulate tumor expansion. Or such molecules could even be designed to activate alternative tumor suppressor genes to shut down the cell cycle of cancer cells. That last goal would effectively shut the door on many cancers and open up new possibilities for cancers now deemed untreatable.

As you can see, the end of cancer relies on a sharpening of vision. So far in this book we have been dealing primarily with a cellular vision. To cure cancer, researchers increasingly will develop a *molecular* vision. Not only will they peer under the lush canopy of DNA but engineer agents to act on the surface of life's molecule, honing their power ever more precisely. According to

Steven Rosenberg, one of the world's leading surgeons and cancer researchers, medical science looks for the slightest crack in a disease and then exploits it. As far as cancer goes, those cracks are occurring at tinier and tinier levels of activity and awareness. Geneticists are working on this level which relies as much on the power of consciousness as technology.

To enhance your consciousness, and enjoy a feeling of empowerment, do this last envisioning exercise on the next page. It is designed to help you identify and hone your power bases so that you can mount one more campaign against cancer's ally: *fear*.

❦ ❦ ❦

Envisioning Exercise

Your Power Bases

Ethics concern choices, and choices can be informed or uninformed. Ethical people are also powerful, not because they have big muscles or wield deadly weapons. They are powerful because like scientists, they try to see the world as it actually is rather than as they would like it to be. To envision the world in such light, they rely on knowledge. They take into account the pertinent facts of a situation and contemplate the range of choices they have that do the least harm to themselves and others. By resolving problems without creating greater ones, they gain confidence in their decision-making abilities. No where in life are these abilities more important than in medical matters, particularly concerning cancer treatment and prevention.

Throughout this book we have stated that knowledge eases fear. After reading this chapter, you have facts that should foster genuine hope for a cancer-free lifestyle in the future. But that future won't arrive soon enough for some individuals. So fear is a daily specter. To combat it, do not yield to the war hammers of cancer thumping your consciousness and making you feel as if no hope remains for you on the immediate horizon. Remember that such a feeling affects attitude, often leading to anger or depression, emotions that thrive on fear. No matter the state of your health, you will be surprised at just how much emotional power you can muster to hone in laser-like on demons that afflict your inner world and attitude.

No one is powerless. Knowledge of that fact alone can go a long way when seeking health care and/or treatment. To realize this, do the exercises below:

I. Identifying Your Power Bases

Most people believe they have only one source of power. Money, for instance. Or influence. The fact is, everyone has more than one power base. To ascertain yours, ask yourself:

- ❖ Am I intellectually powerful? If not, whom can I rely on to inform me about the range of choices that apply to my condition or state of wellness?

- ❖ Do I have access to powerful medical tools or technology? If not, how can I gain such access?

- ❖ Can I communicate powerful ideas to the right medical personnel? If not, how can I gain access to such personnel?

- ❖ What other aspects of my life involve power? Financial base? Political base? Community base? Religious base? Artistic base? Computer base? Science base? Cultural base? Familial base? Others?

II. Honing Your Power Bases

After you have acknowledged your power bases, determine how you have been employing each. Analyze each item on your list. Ask yourself:

- ❖ Have I used this power base in seeking appropriate medical treatment or prevention? If not, how can I?
- ❖ Do I usually exert the appropriate amount of this power to meet each challenge or problem? Or do I usually over- or underestimate situations? When applied to medical care, what are the consequences of over- or underuse of this power?
- ❖ How can I use each power from my various bases to lessen fear, bolster knowledge about cancer, acquire better medical treatment, improve my wellness, and enhance my attitude?

III. Making a Power Collage

Throughout this book you have been asked to use creativity and art as a means to combat fear. This exercise should produce your most treasured work: a power collage representing your best self. To begin the artistic process, ask yourself:

- Were there times in my life when I used one particular power base precisely, appropriately, and effectively?

- How did that moment of accomplishment make me feel? Confident? Proud? Self-assured? Wise? Loving?

After you have reflected on answers to these questions, you should mediate deeply, as you learned in the first chapter. We have come full circle now. Take a deep breath and relax, close your eyes and let your mind lapse to a blank screen in your mind. Let images dissolve on this screen, representing your finest moments and/or accomplishments. If you have enjoyed a good education, say, then remember the pinnacle of your academic career. If you have profited via business or experience, remember scenes of your proudest attainments. This is your collage. Conjure what you will. When you have a clear image, freeze it and then describe it in detail in your personal journal.

Now make a collage. You can draw it yourself on canvas or poster board or describe it to a loved one so that she or he can do that for you. Or you can ask for old magazines and cut out photos and advertisements to reconstruct images similar to ones you have noted in your journal. Or again, ask a loved one to do this for you. You can do the same creative work using a computer and electronic images. In any case, arrange images representing each power base in a design on the canvas, poster, or computer screen.

This is your "Power Collage," representing your best self. When fear strikes, take it out and contemplate the images and draw sustenance from your inner strengths. Celebrate them.

By identifying and honing your power bases, you will assail daily challenges with the whole of your consciousness. Many challenges, especially medical ones, will be beyond your "power." Arguably, the annihilation of fear isn't.

By envisioning your power bases and recapturing past moments of accomplishment, you will mend the cracks in your consciousness, further eroding fear. To vanquish this enemy, continue learning about your own illness or that of a loved one. The more you search for answers about treatment and prevention, the sooner you will come to trust your own inner visions of wellness.

Finally, the authors of *Living Without Fear* want to thank and congratulate you for journeying with us at the microscopic levels of life. By tapping your creativity, we also hope to have inspired you at the yet unmeasurable levels of consciousness. If you have created works of art and craft doing the envisioning exercises in this book, display them around your "Power Collage." Give yourself the gift of your own private showing, or share your works with loved ones in a celebration of you, who have learned so much about science, ethics, art . . . and, most importantly, love's triumph over fear.

His awards include a National Endowment for the Arts fellowship, a National Endowment for the Humanities grant, and an Ohio Arts Council fellowship, among others. Dr. Bugeja has received several teaching honors, including an AMOCO Foundation Outstanding Teacher Award and the University Professor Award. He holds a doctorate in English from Oklahoma State University and a master's in mass communication from South Dakota State University. Before entering academe, he worked as state editor for United Press International. He teaches ethics and writing at the prestigious E. W. Scripps School of Journalism, Ohio University.

Glossary

Adenoma (pronounced *"ADD-ee-NOME-ah"*): a benign tumor in a secretory gland like the intestine.

Adenoviruses (pronounced *"ADD-no-VIGH-rus-es"*): a virus typically found in mild respiratory infections.

Angiogenesis (pronounced *"AN-jee-oh-JEN-ah-sis"*): the process by which new blood vessels emerge from existing blood vessels.

APC: the "gatekeeper" of the intestinal wall and a gene that produces a vital protein, which when mutated, can lead to uncontrolled cell growth in the colorectal region.

ATP: a simple **Metabolite** that provides phosphates to **Cyclin** Dependent **Kinases** that stimulate the cell cycle and a model for small-molecule "decoys" that would deprive CDKs of phosphates.

Chromosomal Translocation: breakage and errant reconnection of chromosomal fragments, causing mutations and sometimes initiating the cancer process.

COX-2: a vital protein and cell-death inhibitor associated with colorectal cancer and which, when found in overabundance, causes pre-cancerous conditions.

Cyclin (pronounced *"SIGH-klin"*): a "vitamin" protein that binds with the dependent "mechanic" protein, otherwise known as Cyclin Dependent **Kinace** (CDK), to help it turn on action molecules of the cell cycle.

Cyclin D: the gatekeeper known as "the driver," perhaps the most important gatekeeper with respect to the onset of cancer, because it prompts cell division.

Cytokines (pronounced *"SITE-oh-kines"*): natural molecules that speed the maturation of stem cells and intermediate cells, again advancing them to their most useful stage (when treating leukemia), when they can rebuild the blood system most effectively.

Dendritic (pronounced *"den-DRIT-ick"*): "super spy" cells of the immune system, which activate two other vital cells of the body's defensive response: killer and helper cells.

DNA: an extremely long and thin molecule, shaped as a double helix, which transfers genetic characteristics to all life forms.

E2F: the "letter-carrier" protein that delivers messages to activate genes that direct production of the "machine" proteins that replicate cells.

Endostatin (pronounced *"END-oh-STAT-in"*): molecular fragments that stop endothelial cells from forming vascular structures.

Endothelial (pronounced *"END-oh-THEEL-ee-all"*): cells that form blood vessels.

Extra-Cellular Matrix Proteins: the "stuff" that coats the outer surface of many cells, including those of our blood vessels, and which bind to **Integrin** molecules on the surface of embryonic **Endothelial** cells, weaving them into tubular sheets. Extra-cellular matrix proteins also are associated with tumor **Angiogenesis**.

Genome (pronounced *"GEE-nome"*): all the inheritable traits of a living creature.

Granulocyte Macrophage Colony Stimulating Factor (pronounced *"GRAN-yoo-LOW-site MACK-re-fage"*) or GMCSF: a signaling protein that activates spy cells of the immune system, bolstering the body's defensive army of white blood cells.

Homeostasis (pronounced *"HOEM-ee-oh-STAY-sis"*): internal stability, or the state of tissues that maintain constant cell numbers by controlling both the rate of cell cycling and the rate of programmed cell death.

Hyperplasia (pronounced *"HIGH-per-PLAY-she-ah"*): a non-malignant tumor resulting from the over-production of cells.

Integrin: a protein that migrates to the outer surface of **Endothelial** cells, stimulating the self-assembly of tubes, and associated with tumor **Angiogenesis**.

Interleukin 2 (pronounced *"IN-ter-LUKE-in"*) or IL-2: a signaling protein that activates killer cells of the immune system.

Kinase (pronounced *"KAI-nace"*): an enzyme that turns on action proteins of the cell cycle, initiating that chemical reaction by adding a phosphate element to amino acids.

Lymph: the pale fluid associated with the immune system, which bathes bodily tissues and carries off bacteria, viruses, and other particles to the **Nodes**.

Lymphocytes (pronounced *"LIMPH-oh-SITES"*): cells associated with the immune system that proliferate and attack foreign particles carried by **Lymph** to the **Nodes.**

Metabolite (pronounced *"met-AB-oh-lite"*): cellular food.

MF-tricyclic (pronounced *"try-SIGH-klick"*): a molecule mistaken by **COX-2** as a **Metabolite** and used as a decoy in the treatment of colorectal cancer.

Mitochondria (pronounced *"MITE-oh-CON-dree-ah"*): the energy-generating bodies within a cell.

Mutagen (pronounced *"MYOOT-a-jens"*): a substance or agent, such as found in tobacco smoke, known to cause mutations (cellular or genetic damage).

Nodes: a complex network of microscopic "mesh," which impedes the passage of foreign objects carried by **Lymph** of the immune system.

Oncogene (pronounced *"ONK-oh-GENE"*): a cancer-related gene.

p16: one of the four gatekeepers that monitors cell division, known by its atomic weight of 16000.

p53: one of the four gatekeepers that suppresses cell division, known by its atomic weight of 53000.

Phosphorylate (pronounced *"foss-FOR-ah-LATE"*): or spraying phosphates. See **Kinace**.

Polymer (pronounced *"POL-ee-mer"*): a molecular compound used in artificial products like polystyrene and polyester and also found in natural substances, including diamonds and **DNA**.

Protease (pronounced *"PRO-tee-ase"*): any enzyme that can chop other proteins into fragments.

Protease Inhibitor: a drug that inhibits **Protease** (used to inhibit a specific protease in the treatment of HIV disease).

RAS: the protein product of an **Oncogene**, associated with colorectal cancer, directly connected to the cell cycle, and which acts as a "carrier pigeon" by dropping messages spawning the powerful gatekeeper "driver," **Cyclin D**.

Retinoblastoma (pronounced *"re-tin-oh-blas-TOM-a"*) or RB protein: one of the four gatekeepers, called the "guard," which prevents rampant cell division by firmly binding **E2F**, preventing it from delivering its messages to prompt cell division.

Proteosomes (pronounced *"PRO-tee-oh-sohms"*): the protein recycling units of the cell that break proteins into small fragments.

Totipotent (pronounced *"toe-tee-POE-tent"*): a cell that has the potential to become any cell in the body.

Vasculogenesis (pronounced *"VAS-cue-loh-JEN-ah-sis"*): Similar to **Angiogenesis**, the rapid and prolific development of blood vessels during some of the earliest phases of an embryo.

Index

About the Authors

Thomas E. Wagner

Thomas E. Wagner is the Director of the Oncology Research Institute at the Greenville Hospital System Cancer Center in Greenville, South Carolina, and is Distinguished Professor of Molecular Medicine at Clemson University. He is at the forefront of the rapidly expanding field of molecular and cellular biology and the emerging biotechnology industry. While an undergraduate at Princeton University he was actively involved with research in the structure and function of DNA. He also was a pioneer in the biotechnology industry, having founded three successful biotechnology companies—DNX, Inc., Diagnostic Hybrids, Inc., and Progenitor, Inc.—and served as a member of the Office of Technology Assessment for Biotechnology of the U.S. Congress. After completing his Ph.D. at Northwestern University he joined the faculty at Cornell University College of Medicine and the staff of the Sloan-Kettering Institute for Cancer Research. In 1970 he joined the faculty at Ohio

University. Dr. Wagner is best known for being the first scientist to introduce permanent functional foreign genes into higher species when he and his research group at Ohio University generated the world's first transgenic animal in 1980. These seminal experiments served as the basis for the establishment of the Ohio University Edison Institute, for which Dr. Wagner served as founding director. He was also Distinguished Professor of Molecular and Cellular Biology and directed research toward the treatment and solution of Cardiovascular Disease, Cancer, AIDS, and allied viral infections.

Michael Bugeja

Michael Bugeja is a nationally known ethicist and author of some 18 books, including the acclaimed *Living Ethics: Developing Values in Mass Communication*. He is ethics adviser to the President of Ohio University, on the Editorial Board of the peer review *Journal of College and Character*, a founding member of the Institute of Applied and Professional Ethics, and creator of the award-winning "Your PATH at Ohio" program, emphasizing personal accountability, trust, and honor. Dr. Bugeja also is president of Character Education Inc., a company that conducts ethics presentations and does consulting work for corporations and educational institutions. Dr. Bugeja is a frequent source about media and applied ethics, interviewed by such outlets as *Fox News, CBS Radio Network, Newsday, American Journalism Review*, and *The Chronicle of Higher Education*. His writings and poems have appeared in a variety of publications, including *Harper's, Word & World, Editor & Publisher, Quill*, and *Journalism Quarterly*.